The Politics of Pain

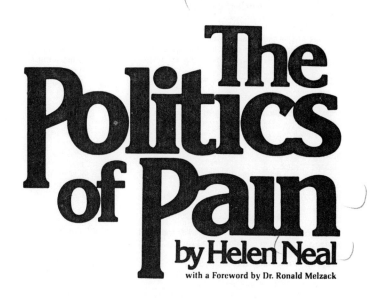

The Politics of Pain

by Helen Neal

with a Foreword by Dr. Ronald Melzack

McGraw-Hill Book Company

New York . St. Louis . San Francisco . Düsseldorf . Mexico . Toronto

Book design by Judy Allan.

1 2 3 4 5 6 7 8 9 0 B P B P 7 8 3 2 1 0 9 8

Library of Congress Cataloging in Publication Data

Neal, Helen.
The politics of pain.
Bibliography: p.
Includes index.
1. Pain. I. Title.
RB127.N43   616'.047   78–6168
ISBN 0–07–046140–6

The author gratefully acknowledges her indebtedness to the following publishers, journals, newspapers, authors, and other copyright owners for their kind permission to quote excerpts:
Academic Press, Inc., and Richard Sternbach, author of *Pain Patients: Traits and Treatment;* Barrie and Jenkins, *The Wild Analyst* by Carl M. Grossman and Sylvia Grossman; Calder & Boyars Ltd., *Medical Nemesis* by Ivan Illich; The Dial Press, *Occult Medicine Can Save Your Life* by C. Norman Shealy with Arthur S. Freese; Little, Brown and Co., and Norman R. Bernstein, author of *Emotional Care of the Facially Burned and Disfigured;* Arnold J. Mandell, author of *The Nightmare Season;* McGraw-Hill Book Company, *Ten Fingers for God* by Dorothy Clarke Wilson; *Medical Times* and Thomas P. Hackett, author of the article "Pain and Prejudice"; *Office Hours: Day and Night* by Janet Travell, M.D., copyright © 1968 by Janet Travell, M.D., reprinted by arrangement with The New American Library, Inc., New York, N.Y.; *The New England Journal of Medicine,* December 18, 1975, Vol. 293, No. 25, page 1320, "Cancer! Alarm! Cancer!" by F. J. Ingelfinger; *Nursing Outlook,* "Pain Assessment on an Orthopedic Ward" by Carolyn L. Wiener, and "Pain: An Organizational-Work-Interactional Perspective" by A. Strauss, S. Y. Fagerhaugh, and B. Glaser; W. B. Saunders Co., *Intractable Pain,* Vol. 2 by Mark Mehta; *Pediatric Nursing* and Margo McCaffery, author of the article "Pain Relief for the Child"; Simon & Schuster, *I Write As I Please* by Walter Duranty; The Society of Authors on behalf of the Bernard Shaw Estate, *Prefaces by Bernard Shaw;* Symposia Specialists, *Current Concepts in the Management of Chronic Pain—"Pro Dolore"* edited by Pierre L. LeRoy, Symposia Specialists, Inc., P.O. Box 610397, Miami, Florida, 33161; *Washington Post,* article in May 11, 1976, issue by Mark Asher, and article in August 31, 1977, issue by Leonard Shapiro; *Washington Star,* article in March 21, 1976, issue by Cristine Russell, and article in the November 9, 1977, issue by Jack W. Germond and Jules Witcover; Congressman Jim Wright, author of *You and Your Congressman.*

In memory of my brother John Richard Neal

Contents

Author's Preface

"Is she a doctor?" the physician asked my friend who, merely to make cocktail party conversation, had told him I was writing a book about pain. When my friend replied that I did not have an M.D. degree, the physician shrugged and turned his attention to his martini.

Crusaders, at least up to now, have never been required to hold advanced degrees in the subjects they espouse. More pertinent to advocacy are indignation, conviction, and a certain set of the will. Somewhere beneath their armor, most crusaders bear the mark of a personal experience, an indelible emotional shock.

Mine came in 1964 when my brother John called from Chicago to tell me he had cancer of the tongue. A shattering diagnosis for anyone, but especially for a crackerjack salesman whose success depended not only on the quality of his merchandise, but on his ability to talk about it. Refusing to succumb to cancer terror, he was determined to run his business, and that meant almost constant traveling, flying from one major city to another.

His treatment got off to a bad start when excessive radiation severely burned his mouth and neck. The codeine prescribed for pain relief by the doctor was totally inadequate. My brother asked me to find out at the National Institutes of Health if there was a more effective analgesic that would control the pain without slowing him down.

At that time, I was a medical science writer at the National Institutes of Health (hereinafter NIH), the federal government's major medical research complex, an enclave of hundreds of scientists. What I found out from NIH pharmacologists and medicinal chemists was of no help to my brother. The consensus was that under the circumstances, codeine, an old standby, was as good an analgesic as any and it was unlikely that anything better would come along for some time, years maybe. Analgesic research, it seemed, was intellectually unexciting to scientists and politically a "downer," of no interest to NIH officials who reflected the cure orientation of the medical profession.

The man who could explain those anomalies and much more besides was Dr. John J. Bonica, world authority on pain, head of the anesthesiology department at the University of Washington, and founder and director of the university's famous pain clinic. We met during the filming of scenes at the pain clinic for an NIH film I was supervising. Dr. Bonica, for personal and professional reasons, had made an evangelical issue of chronic pain, had tried to convince Public Health Service officials and the medical profession that chronic pain was epidemic in America. But he had made little headway. By the time we had finished filming the pain clinic sequences, I was thoroughly committed to Dr. Bonica's cause.

Soon after my return to NIH, my brother John died quite suddenly when a blood vessel, eroded by cancer, hemorrhaged. In the three years since he had first told me about his cancer, he had kept going, crisscrossing the country, resisting mutilating surgery, and never free from pain. With the approval of my director, Dr. Frederick L. Stone, I wrote *Pain*, a brochure that gave an overview of pain, its prevalence, its myths, cultural and ethnic influences on our perception of it, ancient treatment methods, and the need for research in its mechanisms and treatment. Reviewed by Dr. Bonica in manuscript, *Pain* was published in 1968 and, for a simple little information brochure, stirred up a totally unexpected response. Suddenly, people were writing blindly to a government agency (the brochure was anonymous), pouring out incredible stories of suffering: wives dying of cancer, mothers and fathers enduring frightful pain in nursing homes, sisters immobilized by the pain of arthritis. They were heartrending appeals for help in alleviating the pain of members of their families whom physicians were unable to help.

Some physicians were affronted by the publication though it gave no suggestions for the treatment of pain. Several physicians wrote to their congressmen and to the Secretary of Health, Education, and Welfare demanding in rather unprofessional language to know by what authority a government agency presumed to issue a publication on the subject of pain. One physician enclosed a copy of the Constitution of the United States and challenged the Secretary to show wherein the Constitution sanctioned such a publication.

Dentists, however, responded quite differently, their state and county associations ordering thousands of copies. Television and radio commentators used it as a source for broadcast features. According to the producer of an hour-long television documentary, based in part on the brochure, the response to the program was the biggest the network had ever had to a documentary. There was no doubt about the great public interest in pain, but insulated health officialdom continued to overlook evidence it did not wish to see.

In a sense, I had shot my bolt with the publication and when Dr. Stone left NIH in 1968, chances of launching a coordinated pain research program went with him. My interest in pain was well known among my colleagues, many of whom became part of an informal research team, clipping and sending me items about pain, notes about articles, books, and meetings. For want of an official focal point, I became a repository for information about pain and a resource for people outside the NIH calling for help, voices of desperation, unforgettable accounts of unrelieved pain, of being abandoned by physicians. The most I could do for them was to listen and empathize, for there were no pain clinics in the Washington, D.C. area, not even a pain control specialist at the comprehensive cancer center.

But in the mid-1970s there was an explosion of interest and activity in the field of pain. Some influences were easily pinpointed; others were deeper and more subtle, philosophical in nature, like the subject of human rights being extended to include the dying and their right to die comfortably, free from intractable pain. Debate over the Melzack-Wall theory of pain mechanisms, first published in 1965, had heated up in an unseemly fashion, attracting attention like a fistfight at a garden party. Pain clinics, a handful in 1975, had increased to more than 300 two years later, their numbers steadily increasing. Behavioral scientists were reporting on astonishing success in adapting laboratory techniques of modifying behavior to the clinical problem of managing chronic pain. Neurosurgeons, disillusioned by the ephemeral results of pain relief through surgery, were applying their knowledge to developing other solutions. Specialists in the management of pain were getting together in the United States and Europe to talk about developments in basic and clinical pain research, and new diagnostic and treatment methods. In 1974, under Dr. Bonica's leadership, the International Association for the Study of Pain was established and the following year held its first international congress. Attending meetings on pain in America and Europe, listening to the same people, seeing the same names on the programs, it seemed to me that on the pain circuit, enthusiastic as the scientists were about their research, they were primarily interested in talking about it to each other, a propensity, I must emphasize, by no means limited to scientists in the field of pain research. Scientific and medical meetings are essentially hermetic ends in themselves, distinguished more by professional and social camaraderie than by any urge to spread word of the latest findings beyond the meeting room.

To be sure, proceedings are sometimes published and with that, organizers of the meetings consider their communications duty done. But how many physicians in private practice, confronted daily by patients with chronic pain, can find answers to their treatment problems in published proceedings that are usually outrageously high-priced and always smorgasbords of unevaluated research findings, each report given equal status without any clue for separating significant from inconsequential research?

As for sufferers and their families, they are merely abstractions at professional meetings. In all the meetings I have attended, I have never seen a pain patient on the platform to tell his or her side of the story. By 1975, it seemed to me that advances in pain management warranted direct communication with pain patients and their families. Though for one reason or another they would not write it themselves, scientists and health practitioners I interviewed encouraged me to write the book on pain and generously shared their knowledge and ideas.

I wrote this book chiefly to let people in on the numerous choices there are now for controlling pain, where to get help, and their right, even obligation as medical consumers, to participate in decisions regarding pain treatment. Beyond that, I wanted to share some of the fascination of the subject of pain itself, its functions and mysteries, its strange rewards and uses, its religious, psychological, and cultural aspects, and man's search through the ages for the magic cure. I also felt it important to disclose some of the political impediments to research in pain control methods, the deplorable pain management policies in hospitals, and the medical profession's general disregard for chronic pain in children.

It is my hope that activist readers will work for changes in pain management systems in hospitals and nursing homes, and that they will impress on their congressmen the need for a national, coordinated program of pain research, treatment, and training.

In personal and public ways, for ourselves and others we love, we can now control the silent epidemic of pain.

Washington, D.C., 1978

Foreword

The field of pain research and therapy has suddenly come alive—full of new controversy and renewed fascination. The simple-minded answers of the past are being critically examined, and new questions are constantly being raised to challenge the scientist. Most exciting of all, important advances in research and theory are being translated into effective clinical techniques.

Helen Neal has captured the excitement that comes with the explosion of knowledge in a new field of medicine. The relief of pain is probably the oldest of human medical endeavors. But only recently have physicians and scientists come to recognize that chronic pain is not merely a symptom of some disease or injury but is a major medical problem in its own right. Severe chronic pain is profoundly disabling. It is a pathological process that deserves special attention, a sympathetic concern from physicians, and new, distinctive approaches aimed at alleviating it.

When chronic pain—such as low back pain or persistent headaches—disables a young worker for years, decades, even a lifetime, the cost to society in compensation benefits is enormous. There is also the cost of hospital care, physicians, consultants, drugs, operations, and so forth. The Politics of Pain, therefore, is an appropriate title for this book. Pain is not merely a medical problem, it is also an economic problem involving billions of dollars. And thus it is a political concern because decisions have to be made at a variety of government levels on the sources and uses of those funds. The loss in time at work and the loss of an effective person at home are costly to the sufferer, the immediate family, and society in general. But most important is the suffering patient, and it is for this person that Helen Neal has written this book.

The book will play an important role in teaching people to recognize pain as a major medical problem. It is relevant for the patient as well as for the physician. Our pill-popping culture, with promises of total pain relief, has led patients and physicians to expect that a given drug or therapy should be effective for *all* pain in *all* patients. No such therapy has been found and there is no reason to believe it will be. The patient who is told that he must learn to live with pain usually concludes that the physician is incompetent and visits doctor after doctor searching for perfect control of pain.

Medical practitioners must accept partial blame for this state of affairs. The persistence of outmoded pain theories in medical school teaching and practice has sometimes led to treatments that further complicate the patient's condition. After countless ineffective treatments, the patient is often dismissed as a malingerer or a neurotic. Small wonder that such patients are depressed, resentful, and anxious.

Helen Neal has written an important, useful book. She has written it with compassion and understanding as well as with the fervor of a person who has seen someone she loves die in pain. She is committed to her cause and does an excellent job in achieving her goal. By presenting an up-to-date account of the new kinds of treatment for pain and by directing people in pain to the major hospitals and pain centers at which they are available, Helen Neal has provided an extremely valuable service to the millions of sufferers—and potential sufferers—of chronic pain. Her book comes, moreover, at a remarkably opportune time—when the breakthroughs are occurring and new approaches are being developed, including electrical stimulation of peripheral nerves, acupuncture, and new psychiatric, pharmacological, and neurosurgical approaches. It reflects all of the excitement of a field undergoing rapid change— and, as the pieces of the puzzle of pain are seen to fall into place, it provides the pleasure and excitement that comes with growing insight into a major problem.

Ronald Melzack, Ph.D.
Director of Pain Research,
Montreal General Hospital
Professor of Psychology,
McGill University
Montreal, Quebec, Canada

1 | the Politics of Pain

At any DAR convention, Mrs. Bessie D. would blend inconspicuously with the other matronly, well-dressed, soft-spoken women. There's nothing about her that marks her out as a drug addict. Yet, she is. Like thousands of other women and men living a kind of half-life with low back pain, she's medically addicted to drugs. For sixteen years she has gone desperately from one doctor to another, has had seven back operations, always expecting the next surgeon will cure the pain. She worries about the debts. But pain and worry about money are at times overshadowed by the realization that, a respected, church-going woman, she is a drug addict, a dependence that began years ago when her doctor, unable to find anything physically wrong with her, had given her pain relievers to keep her "comfortable." She could tell he wasn't interested in her any more as a patient; he merely renewed her drug prescription when she went to him, but never bothered to check her heart or blood pressure. Only surgeons took any notice of her. The first operation brought some relief, but only for a few months. The other operations didn't help much either. And by that time, she was trapped. Pain had become the "beloved symptom," the

1

arbiter of her life. She had joined the ranks of the medical rejects.

In this era of anxiety and chronic diseases, pain surfaces as a major medical and psychological problem. It is not known for certain how many Americans suffer from it, but estimates run as high as from 35 to 40 million people. Of the 21 million arthritics, some 19 million endure pain that ranges from mild to totally disabling. Hundreds of thousands endure the excruciating torment of terminal cancer pain. Some 7 million men and women have low back pain. Losses from work productivity from this disability are calculated at about $14 to $15 billion a year. One hundred thousand severely burned victims suffer not only from the burns themselves, but also from almost unbearable treatments, the dressing changes, and the horrendous "scrubbing and tubbing."

As yet no yardstick has been devised for measuring the human suffering, the suicides, divorces, ruined careers, mental breakdowns, and bankruptcy. Men and women, diligent and thrifty, are pauperized by medical costs for operations, medications, and hospital care. Among the 32 million disabled Americans, almost 12 million are severely disabled from injuries, disease, or birth defects. Thirty-five percent of those who are 20 to 64 years of age suffer musculoskeletal disorders in which pain can reasonably be considered a major factor. Millions of former workers, a large percentage of them suffering from low back pain, collect billions in disability payments. From $40 to $50 billion is the estimated cost of pain in health costs, loss of work productivity, litigation, and compensation payments.

To sufferers of chronic disease and pain, drained emotionally, physically, even financially, forsaken by doctors, and a nuisance to their families, the lure of the quack is irresistible. He never tells them: "There's nothing more I can do for you." He solaces them with promises of magical cures that sometimes occur, not because the costly pills or mystifying machines work miracles, but because what the quack really sells is faith and hope. Desperate Americans every year give $2½ billion to quacks for cancer cures and the relief of arthritic pain. Traditionally, doctors divide pain into two categories: acute and chronic. In their lexicon, acute pain is sharp, an urgent signal that something has gone wrong, some organ is not functioning properly, or a muscle is sprained or a bone broken. It usually subsides when the cause is cured. This is the pain doctors have been trained to diagnose and treat expertly. When it comes to diagnosing and treating chronic pain, they are less adept. They become frustrated, irritated, and eager to get rid of the patients. In hospitals, people who have chronic, undiagnosed pain are labeled "chrons," the neurotics, complainers, even fakers. If a doctor cannot diagnose your pain, he sends you to someone else or doses you with painkillers. Trained to cure, and usually very good at that, doctors derive their professional satisfaction from seeing a patient get well, restored to health and activity. Learned optimists about acute pain, when confronted by persistent pain that seems to have no physical cause, they dismiss patients with: "It's all in your head." Or prescribe addictive drugs.

A type of pain that is not much talked about in medical circles is that caused by new diagnostic and treatment techniques. In burn units, screaming, crying, yelling accounts in large part for the high turnover of staff. The encouraging statistics of survival rates among children who have leukemia conceal the anguish caused by the treatment, the frequent painful sticking of their fingers for blood samples and, far worse, bone marrow aspiration, a procedure in which hip or breastbones are punctured and the marrow in the bone drawn out by a syringe. Leukemic children endure this type of suffering for years, several days a week during intensive treatment, and if there is a remission of the disease, every few months. Modern medicine has given us a new type of chronic pain, but not the methods for controlling it.

Reverence for life is a characteristic of democracy. The mere extension of life in America is looked upon as one of the great scientific achievements of our century. All babies, regardless of how horrible their birth defects, must be saved, bodies mangled in car wrecks patched up. Modern medicine does its lifesaving job magnificently and sends its grotesqueries into society. Machines feed the helpless, fragile aged, staving off death. At all costs, death must be defied.

What we haven't yet got around to is greater concern for alleviating the suffering of the living. Pain, a very private, personal affair, has had no official spokesman. Perhaps for that reason and because it has been with us since the beginning of time, it has been largely disregarded by doctors and scientists. No one, except the person experiencing it, doubts the value of pain as a warning of something amiss, but its value depends on the availability of means for correcting it. Until a hundred years ago a king, in a medical sense, was no better off than a peasant. The "warning" pains of a rupturing appendix merely doubled them up in agony. The peasant in his dying moments fared better than the king, who was set upon by physicians who bled and purged him.

People through the ages, with the help of theologians, have somehow found ways of dealing with continuing pain when nothing could be done to alleviate it. One endured. But in our time the passive virtue of endurance is out of fashion. A new self-consciousness, an awareness of human rights, demands that something be done, batters against a wall of scientific and medical indifference.

How does one account for this indifference? A partial explanation comes from Dr. Lucius Sinks, oncologist at Georgetown University Hospital in Washington, D.C., who told me that scientists "don't want to get mired in some line of investigation that is so complex and unlikely to have important payoffs and clear-cut findings. Things have changed since the days when scientists at Cambridge and Oxford could steal away and hide out in some dingy laboratory and follow their particular interest. No one was breathing down their backs for results, demanding some advance in knowledge that would look good on the application for grant renewal.

"But things are different now. The scientist is out in the open, exposed to constant review, competing for money that gets less and less. Pain is a very difficult area to study. It's complicated by all sorts of factors that are hard to measure, very personal reactions all tied up with the way people have been brought up, what they expect from life, and their problems of the moment. Scientists have tended to leave the subject to those they consider the spooks, the hypnotists and alchemists."

As chief of the division of Pediatric and Adolescent Oncology at the hospital, Dr. Sinks is especially concerned with the pain of children who have cancer. Their extended survival period, he said, "creates a type of chronic pain, sometimes from the cancer, sometimes from the treatment, sometimes from both. We're in a new period of medicine now. The situation will be the strongest argument. As medicine and science prolong the lives of cancer patients, there will be a prolonging of the period of chronic pain. For that much longer period, there will have to be new and better methods of controlling pain."

Most scientists agree with Dr. Sinks's appraisal of pain as being complex and unlikely to have payoffs. One scientist put it even more simply: "Pain is a mess." That, however, is not entirely the reason scientists back off from it. Genetics is a mess, too. But genetics is "pure" science, one of the basic sciences that are seedbeds of Nobel Prizes and nesting grounds for elitists unwilling to accommodate their own professional aims to public needs, the scientists who, in and out of government, champion "the scientist's right to know" at public expense. They dominated the policies of the federal government's largest health research agency, the National Institutes of Health, until it lost its scientific virginity in the Oval Office of the White House when Lyndon Johnson summoned the directors of the institutes and ordered them to sponsor more research that would benefit the public which footed the bill. Across the nation, word flashed from their bureaucratic counterparts at the National Institutes of Health to scientists, instructing them to put in their grant applications something about their research being "health related."

It is questionable whether the political use of that phrase did much to reroute research into areas more closely related to the major health problems of the nation. Rarely do civil servants prod scientists or even encourage them to shift their research into other areas. The exception occurs when the officials themselves are prodded by the Congress or the White House.

An example of this occurred after President Nixon returned from China and indicated his interest in acupuncture. Top officials of the National Institutes of Health jumped to attention. An expression of interest by the White House is tantamount to marching orders. Several officials sought out a scientist of Chinese ancestry whose Chinese name would look impressive on reports. He was pressured into putting aside his own research in order to investigate acupuncture. Dependent on the National Institutes of Health for his research funds, he organized a study of acupuncture. In the midst of it, Nixon departed from the White House. High-level scientific interest in acupuncture plummeted. The scientist with the Chinese name learned firsthand a great deal about politics of science.

Scientists go where the money is. "Not the really good ones!" say the elitists. Yet it's the elitists who protest to the Congress and the press that the National Cancer Institute with its billions is enticing first-rate scientists from equally important areas of science. Basil O'Connor, when president of the Infantile Paralysis Foundation, *demanded* a polio vaccine, paid for it, and got it from topflight scientists.

Another reason pain control is in the medical and scientific broom closet is that there isn't any money in it. Federal and voluntary health agencies raise their money—the former from the Congress, the latter directly from the public—on promises of cure. Pain, in fund-raising parlance, is a "downer." Neither the Arthritis Foundation nor the American Cancer Society, raising money for the cure of diseases in which pain is inherent, mentions pain control as a research objective. And neither agency supports pain research. Practically, as sophisticated fund-raising agencies, they are wise to steer clear of the subject of pain in their fund-raising literature. "Give to cure cancer in your lifetime," misleading as that slogan is, has raised so much money that the American Cancer Society has an embarrassing surplus.

National voluntary health agencies are the bureaucratic sisters of governmental bureaucracies. Hand in hand, they go to the public trough for money. They are equally adept at manipulating public fears and statistics. The Public Health Service, for the same reasons as the voluntary health agencies, has shied away from the topic of pain. Old China hands know that members of Congress respond to drama, show, crises, and their constituents. Ameliorating pain, making life more endurable for chronic sufferers and the terminally ill, is not the kind of thing that rallies votes or puts bronze name plaques on the walls of hospitals and medical centers. Understandably, federal health officials, reading with exquisite sensibility the congressional mind and heart, when budget hearings take place, stick with the "cure" propaganda and well-documented promises. Consequently, the Congress has been kept in ignorance of the magnitude of the pain problem, its extent and incalculable costs, and what should be done about it.

The powerful congressional committees set the course for health programs in a hit-or-miss fashion. The prevalence or gravity of a disease is not necessarily the guide to their decisions. A lot depends on what is wrong with significant numbers of their own constituents. In a national context, the incidence of a disease may be minuscule, but if it affects a vocal constituency, congressmen see to it that funds are allocated for research on its causes and ways of treating it. Cooley's anemia is an example. Prevalent in the Mediterranean area, in the United States there are some 2,400 cases. Over the years, millions of dollars have been allotted for the study of Cooley's anemia through the influence of a congressman in whose district reside many voters whose origins are in the Mediterranean area.

As a consequence of the "pet disease" policy, priorities in health programs are constantly revised. Emphasis on certain diseases and disabilities surges and ebbs as congressmen and presidents come and go. Public health officials long ago gave up trying to set priorities and stick to them. They present programs they know will get generous appropriations. The subject of pain has been discreetly ignored.

And the press has not been of help in this matter. They, who should be the watchdogs, critics, commentators, and alerters, write mostly about "curative medicine." Medical and science reporting burgeoned after the Russians launched the first satellite and American science leaped to catch up. In the 1960s the medical and scientific press developed a fine corps of journalists. But in the 1970s as competition forced newspapers out of business, medical and science writers were among the first to lose their jobs. Some went into other fields. Many medical writers went to journals and newsletters published by pharmaceutical companies. Those who survived on newspapers were hardly in a position to be watchdogs and critics. Editors demanded news stories of exciting new "cures," no matter how flagrantly premature the research might be. Dr. James E. Turner in an article[1] on research sensationalism says it "provides grist for the mills of the lay press, for the public-relations directors of grant-seeking medical schools, for the many beholden investigators who must deliver politically useful health publicity in order to continue their grants from year to year.... It encourages public and Presidential belief that medical research can produce instant miracle breakthroughs." But breakthroughs are what editors want, stories that say in essence: "New Hope for the Dead!"

Harold M. Schmeck, Jr., New York Times medical science writer, told a group of neuroscientists who had just given a session for the press on the scientific bafflement and frustration of pain research that if he had filed a story that day on the subject, his editor would be faced with choosing stories on the Middle East, a congressional battle, and a story: "Neuroscientists Say Nature of Pain Is Not Entirely Clear."

Except in feature stories, pain lacks editorial appeal. Medical journals, largely supported by advertisements for pharmaceutical products, emphasize the control of pain by drugs. Designed for physicians, these journals, filled with ads and articles about analgesics, do very little to educate physicians on alternative methods of pain control.

Medical journalists are indentured to their governmental and academic sources of information. If they write a critical story about an agency or an official, the sources penalize them in subtle ways, cutting off access to information, refusing interviews. Consequently these journalists in a tight job market rely on news releases, press conferences arranged by health officials to disseminate their own propaganda, and interviews which can be guaranteed to be friendly. In this custodial news atmosphere, medical writers rarely dig for stories and expose issues officials are not interested in promoting. The problem of pain is one such issue, much written about in features that explore its mysteries but that rarely mention the failure of the medical profession or governmental or private health agencies to recognize the extent of the problem.

One further stumbling block in making progress in pain control is the federal government's politicized drug addiction program launched in 1974 by former President Nixon—"The War of the Poppies." John Ehrlichman, former White House aide, put this "war" in political perspective when he testified before a Senate committee in 1976. Narcotic suppression, he said, "is a very sexy political issue. It usually has high media visibility. Parents are worried about narcotics. They listen to a politician talking about drug suppression when they tune him out on the energy problem. Therefore the White House often wants to be involved in the narcotics problems, even when it doesn't need to be."

The "War of the Poppies" had little effect on illicit drug traffic but enormous impact on medical care. Foreign countries, Turkey in particular, bribed not to grow poppies from which opium and its many derivatives come, gladly took the millions. But the peasants, whose livelihood depended on the poppies, continued to grow them.[2]

Nixon's customary allies, the chieftains of organized medicine, arose to protest his drive against the production of opium. Morphine and its derivatives are essential for controlling acute and chronic pain. Pharmaceutical companies, faced with losses in revenues, added their protests to those of the medical profession. A scientist who courageously spoke out against White House policy was Dr. William T. Beaver of Georgetown University. He publicly questioned whether the suppression of opium growth would reduce the availability of illicit heroin enough to justify the adverse effect on patient care and medical research. The United States policy, he said, "is likely to have a substantial world-wide impact on certain aspects of medical practice, in particular the management of pain, and on several major areas of biomedical research." The White House soft-pedaled its publicity on suppressing opium production abroad. Morphine supplies continued to flow into hospitals and pharmacies.

The government's drug abuse prevention and law enforcement program, involving at least fifteen federal agencies and billions of dollars since 1974, has failed to stop drug peddling or its consumption. Its greatest impact has been on millions of chronic pain sufferers.

Physicians, intimidated by the sinister climate surrounding the war on drug addiction, "undermedicate" their hospitalized patients who have persistent, intense pain, many of them hopelessly ill.

Heroin, considered by many physicians and scientists to be the most effective of all pain relievers, has not been available for medical use in the United States, though widely used in England and other countries. It is a fast-acting drug that does not cause the respiratory problems common with morphine, or the constipation, or the depression. A scientist, world-renowned for his research on analgesics, told me that if he were dying from a painful cancer, heroin would be his "drug of choice." Besides its effectiveness as a painkiller, it lifts the spirit and, he said, that's something a dying person is entitled to.

Though heroin is readily obtainable on street corners in every city despite the government's massive efforts to prevent its sale, it is denied to terminally ill patients who have cancer. A result of the government's huge publicity campaign, rivaling a great war propaganda effort, is that, in the public mind, the word *heroin* triggers fear and agitation, like the word *rape*. Yet heroin damages the body and the mind far less than alcohol and compared to alcohol is a minor social problem. The cost of alcoholism in the United States is estimated to be $15 billion a year. In 1977, there were 1 million alcoholic teenagers.

The focus of the government's anti-drug addiction and law enforcement programs is 500,000 heroin addicts. Oddly, those bureaucracies are not concerned with the estimated 2 million "chippers," occasional users of heroin who somehow manage to control their habit and apparently do not have to resort to crime to support it. In the public and bureaucratic mind, the typical heroin addict is a skinny young black, spaced out, slumped in a refuse-strewn doorway in a big city slum. If caught with heroin, he is arrested. Governmental agencies run a few treatment centers where they "cure" these addicts with another addicting drug, methadone. The root of the problem, the ghetto life, gangs, despair, is attacked by a handful of overworked guidance counselors, social workers, and group leaders whose efforts are supported by a pittance.

The failure of the federal anti-drug addiction program is due in part to its profound cynicism. In Washington, D.C., which has one of the highest per capita incidences of heroin addiction in the country, when cuts were made in the local budget of the Office of Human Development—while officials were lavishly redecorating their private offices—the administrator, with public tears, announced the closing of several drug treatment centers. Hundreds of addicts seeking treatment were turned away. Hundreds already in the treatment program joined them. Not one federal agency involved in the anti-drug addiction program offered emergency funds to keep the treatment centers open. Nor was there a public outcry. Nor did newspaper editors castigate local and federal governmental agencies for this outrageous demonstration of the basic cynicism of the war on drug addiction. But when narcotics agents capture a few pounds of heroin, efficient publicity machines flood the press with stories and photographs.

One minute the federal government was pressuring Mexico to crack down on drug traffickers and the next it was pressuring them to return Americans jailed on drug charges who were badgering their congressmen and families with pitiful stories about how uncomfortable Mexican jails are. And what did the Congress that has voted billions to stop the drug trade in this country do about those pleas? In November 1977, the Foreign Relations Committee came up with an unprecedented treaty, arranging for an exchange of American and Mexican prisoners. About 250 young Americans, mostly jailed on hard drug charges, would be returned to the United States to finish out their terms in more comfortable jails. An added advantage for those Americans is that in this country, they will be eligible for parole. The Mexican government, very serious about its anti-drug program, does not parole those convicted of possessing hard drugs.

The Congress authorized $1,700,000 for the first exchange, all expenses of the prisoners' travel to be paid by American taxpayers. Thoughtfully, the treaty provides for future trips from Mexican jails to homeland prisons by allocating $1,600,000 for 1979 and the same amount for 1980. The amounts, it should be pointed out, include transportation, counseling, and the cost of imprisonment in the United States, estimated at $25,000 a prisoner for one year. A further point is that parents of the young Americans imprisoned in Mexico on drug charges used considerable leverage on congressmen to get their children out of those tough Mexican jails.

The first contingent of those convicted heroin traffickers and marijuana smugglers rescued by the American government arrived in San Diego shortly before Christmas, 1977. Relatives and friends greeted them with banners, flags, and balloons. Contributing to the festive spirit were the new red, white, and blue uniforms the American government had provided the young prisoners.

About the time negotiations were going on for the return of those young addicts and pushers, their less influential counterparts in Harlem were the object of official ceremonial attention of sorts. Diplomats from twenty-two countries that export large quantities of narcotics were taken in buses with police escort through the streets of the ghetto where they were shown the human wreckage of the drug trade. Men idling on the streets stared back at the diplomats, laughed, and made an occasional obscene gesture. The purpose of the tour was to wring the hearts and consciences of the representatives of those countries from which vast amounts of narcotics come. The diplomats could not have failed to be impressed on several counts. One, that a government so devoted to human rights would degrade its own people by putting them on display, much as a century ago men and women were displayed in madhouses. And, on another count, the diplomats must have wondered about how things really are in the richest democracy in the world where so many of its people live in what look like war-ravaged buildings.

The government's anti-drug addiction program might be dismissed as a grotesque political game but for its indirect penalties on medical practice and scientific advances in pain control. The criminal aura surrounding narcotic drugs subtly deters many scientists from undertaking analgesic research. The carefully nurtured social stigma attached to narcotics and marijuana rubs off on those who would use them in experiments for medical purposes. Besides the medicinal value of heroin, long established in medical practice in foreign countries, other drugs, marijuana and LSD, have proved beneficial in studies of patients with terminal cancer. But only a few dogged scientists have been willing to put up with the governmental restrictions and oversight that hover around scientific experiments in their use.

The stigma spreads to the development of synthetic analgesics. Knowing that official interest is not primarily on the pain-relieving efficacy of the analgesic, but on its addictive potential, few scientists are willing to devote their careers to developing synthetic painkillers. It takes as many as seven years to develop some synthetic analgesics from the initial experiments in transposing molecules, trying different combinations, testing on animals, controlled studies on patients, and, if the new drug passes all those hurdles, its manufacture and marketing. Years of exacting research can be nullified if a drug, no matter how effective for controlling pain, is highly addictive. Not that addiction potential shouldn't be considered (though most effective synthetic analgesics widely used in medical practice are addictive), but you can understand the reluctance of scientists to go into this line of research. Yet there is a critical need for analgesics specifically for children, and for particular types of pain, cancer, arthritis, and serious burns.

Only the President of the United States could axe through the Gordian knot of bureaucratic restrictions on the use of heroin, marijuana, and LSD in studies of their therapeutic value for terminally ill cancer patients and those undergoing aggressive cancer treatment. President Jimmy Carter did just that in September 1977, in an order to the Department of Health, Education, and Welfare to reassess all drugs, including heroin and marijuana, on "a purely scientific basis not colored by the past history" of governmental policy.

The order was cautiously worded lest the Justice Department's Drug Enforcement Agency and the public get the impression that the President advocated indiscriminate use of heroin. The President's special assistant for health issues, Dr. Peter Bourne, a psychiatrist and author of the policy change, explained to the press that the effectiveness of heroin for pain relief has been demonstrated in Great Britain and dozens of other countries, but in the United States only a few isolated studies of the illicit drug had been carried out.

Writing about the change of policy, Jack W. Germond and Jules Witcover said in the *Washington Star* that the therapeutic use of heroin and marijuana had been prevented by "timidity among both the politicians and the bureaucrats. Few of the former have considered this a rewarding issue on which to get 'out front,' and most of the latter have been understandably cautious in such a political climate."

Medical researchers would be free to conduct studies without fear of harassment. And the authors of the *Washington Star* article concluded: "And, beyond that, what the episode tells us is that changing administrations in Washington can affect people's lives in more ways than is always apparent in our tunnel focus on major issues of the time. For a terminal cancer patient, the availability of heroin can be much more important than the fine print in the energy bill."

Predictably, presidential attention to the plight of terminal cancer patients stirred sudden interest among public health officials in the whole subject of pain, a development that one man had been awaiting for twenty years. For decades he waged a lonely, dogged crusade, speaking at medical and science meetings, writing books and articles, trying to convince physicians, scientists, and Public Health Service officials that pain is epidemic in the United States and that something should be done about it. Dr. John J. Bonica, the world's foremost authority on pain research and treatment, director of the renowned pain clinic at the University of Washington, learned firsthand about pain in an unusual way. He was a professional wrestler, literally wrestling his way through medical school as the Masked Marvel. Thirty years later, injuries from those wrestling matches that paid for his medical education caught up with him. But long before he became a chronic pain sufferer himself, he developed the concept of the multidisciplinary approach to pain management—an array of specialists who focus on the pain problem of each patient. Despite his crusading efforts, Dr. Bonica had made little headway in persuading administrators at the National Institutes of Health to launch a coordinated pain research and training program.

True, the National Institutes of Health and the National Institute on Drug Abuse were funding research in analgesics, anesthesia, and pain mechanisms; but at the time this book was being written in 1977, it was impossible to get an analysis of the total federal effort. Nor was there coordination of the research or priorities for certain areas of pain research. The National Institute on Aging and the National Institute of Child Health and Human Development supported no pain research, yet it would seem those two institutes should have had a primary interest in it. The only institute of the National Institutes of Health with a formalized pain research program was the National Institute of Dental Research, attuned as it is to the major problem in dentistry—public fear that having teeth fixed is going to hurt, a fear that discourages millions of people from going to the dentist until they get a toothache. The National Cancer Institute, with an annual budget of almost a billion dollars, had $600,000 invested in pain research grants and at the same time was spending $6,000,000 on the development of a "safe" cigarette.

Behind almost every institute of the National Institutes of Health you find an advocate, a powerful individual or voluntary agency, or professional association. A sample of these couplings shows: the American Cancer Society/National Cancer Institute; American Heart Association/National Heart and Lung Institute; Arthritis

Foundation/National Institute of Arthritis, Metabolism, and Digestive Diseases (metabolism and digestive diseases were add-ons, each promoted by special-interest groups); and Research to Prevent Blindness/National Eye Institute. These advocates marshal their memberships when Congress holds its budget hearings, recruit distinguished witnesses to appear before the committees, and organize letter-writing campaigns.

The problem of pain needed that kind of organized backing. In 1974, Dr. Bonica and a group of scientists organized the International Association for the Study of Pain, which held its first world congress in Florence, Italy, in 1975. Twice as many participants showed up as had been expected from all over the world—scientists, physicians, psychologists, nurses, therapists. It was evident that advances in the basic and behavioral sciences, discoveries about pain mechanisms, new types of treatment, and the advent of the pain clinic had given the subject of pain a new persona. Some American scientists and physicians felt there should be a national association that would promote coordination of research, evaluation of present treatment methods, and information programs for health professionals and the general public.

In February 1977, Dr. B. Berthold Wolff, pain research scientist at New York University and president of the Eastern USA Regional Chapter of the International Association for the Study of Pain, proposed the establishment of the American Pain Society. The Society was formed in October 1977.

Up to that time, only one federal agency, the Social Security Administration, had officially recognized the pain problem when, in 1976, it authorized Medicare payments for treatment and rehabilitation in pain clinics.

There were few pain clinics at the time, but stimulated by the availability of federal funds, the number of pain clinics increased phenomenally to 330 in 1977.

By whatever name—pain clinics, centers, units—they are the refuge of medical rejects, people whose suffering may be from known or unknown causes, whose doctors have either abandoned them or keep them quiet with heavy doses of analgesics. Some clinics adopt Dr. Bonica's model of focusing on each patient the expertise of neurologists, internists, surgeons, psychologists, nurses, anesthesiologists, therapists, and social workers. Other clinics specialize in one type of pain such as headache or low back pain, while others treat the full range. Some are privately run clinics, others units in hospitals or part of rehabilitation centers. Wherever they are, whatever their specialties, pain clinics are a medical growth industry.

The yeast in pain control movement is the behavioral scientist. In the 1960s these scientists began applying to people with chronic pain the techniques used in laboratory experiments with animals. Psychologists recognized in some patients symptoms of what is now called "pain behavior," patterns built up around the experience of pain in a desperate attempt to cope with it. Unlike physicians, psychologists are not easily put off by personality quirks, idiosyncrasies, faults, and foibles. They are unhampered by a hyped-up attitude toward cure. The nature of their training fosters infinite patience and they are comfortable in long-term relationships with people whose progress toward set goals is likely to be slow and faltering. Not pill-oriented or targets of seductive advertising by pharmaceutical companies, psychologists boldly explore alternatives to drug treatment. They write books and articles about successful techniques of pain control—operant conditioning, biofeedback, hypnosis, group therapy. Enthusiastic investigators, they share, in symbiotic harmony, platforms with neuroscientists, physicians, and surgeons, speaking the new jargon in the new specialty of pain management.

This new specialty relieves physicians from frustration and guilt over their inability to help many of their patients who suffer from chronic pain. Now, without abandoning them, doctors can refer them to professional pain managers.

As yet there are not enough physicians and psychologists specializing in pain management, nor nearly enough pain clinics. That will come only as part of a national, coordinated effort involving federal, professional, and private agencies. The many-faceted approach advocated by Dr. Bonica and others includes:

- A task force to review the status of pain research, treatment, and training
- Coordination of research in governmental, private and academic institutions
- Evaluation of data collected from pain clinics on the effectiveness of different procedures for relieving intractable pain
- A physicians' information center for pain treatment methods
- Evaluation of treatment methods already in use for specific types of pain
- A public information program on pain management alternatives

When physicians and medical scientists get together, they talk a great deal about "the patient" and after you've listened for hours or days, it's easy to forget that "the patient" they're talking about is a real person. It's an 84-year-old woman dying of cancer, trying to conceal her suffering from her grown children gathered at her hospital bedside. And her older son, unable to bear the sight of her suffering, leaving the room and, with tears in his eyes, telling the hospital chaplain that, if it would help his mother, he would have his arm cut off. And its a 53-year-old man who, until his back injury a year before, was a healthy, vigorous construction worker. Now he sits at home in a stupor, overdosed with narcotic analgesics. Ask any nurse in a burn treatment unit about the "noise level," the screaming, sobbing, and groans as dressings are changed on raw flesh. Or what the sounds are like on the cancer ward at three in the morning. Multiplying those sounds of human distress by millions gives some idea of the magnitude and urgency of the pain epidemic in America. There is a solution, not primarily medical, but political.

2 Pain Types

"Where does it hurt?"

"What does it feel like?"

The two questions most frequently asked in medical practice.

Pain is the "great persuader," responsible for 90 percent of visits to doctors. But a curious thing about this persuader is that it isn't always persuasive at the outset. People generally ignore minor aches, intermittent twinges, vague dull discomfort in the stomach or back, even sharp pains in the head. Some people put up with rather intense pain for days, weeks, sometimes months, even years without going to a doctor about it.

Then something happens. A husband walks out on his wife...a son is arrested on marijuana charges... a typist is fired...a middle-aged woman who had considered herself youthful and trendy is given a seat on the bus by a teenager. Pain that had been ignored or stoically endured is perceived all at once as threatening and intolerable. The sufferer seeks medical help. Physicians first look for some physical cause, for instance an ulcer, or gallstones, or an erratic heart. This is the type of pain physicians have been trained to control, diagnose and cure the physical cause. But if physicians are baffled by a patient's persistent pain, can't find any physical reason for it, they become suspicious, annoyed, even hostile.

If a computer medical profile labeled you a "chronic benign patient," you might, if you were an English major, feel understandably flattered. And with some reason, for interpreted literally the phrase means you are habitually gracious and of gentle disposition. But in pain jargon, it means you have a continuous pain of mild character or pain not caused by a deadly disease.

In a field already as confused as a Jackson Pollock painting, the imprecise terms used to describe various types of pain are a major hindrance to communications between physicians and patients and even among pain specialists themselves. Advances in knowledge about pain have outstripped its definitions. In medical schools, students are told there are two types of pain: acute and chronic. Acute pain is defined as "sharp, penetrating and of short duration." Chronic pain, according to textbooks, is any pain that persists for six months or more.

As medical students study diseases, they learn to interpret types of pain as symptoms of disease—the chest pains of angina pectoris, the pain pattern of duodenal ulcers, the "referred" pain of spinal cord diseases. Pain is presented as a clue, not an entity in itself. It is assumed that in medical practice physicians will decode the pain message, find the cause, and cure it. But physicians are not trained in the control of pain for which they can find no physical cause, nor are they taught to distinguish the many types of chronic pain that have in a sense individual personalities.

Even the definition of acute pain as short-lasting is not always accurate. In fact, one reason physicians become frustrated and irritated by patients is that their "acute pain" doesn't stop when, according to the textbooks, it should do so. It is at that point that many physicians tell patients "There's nothing more that I can do for you," dismissing them at the very stage in the pain process when alternative methods of pain control should be instituted, before pain behavior takes hold.

The term *chronic pain* lumps together at least five types of chronic pain that should be specially treated:

- Chronic pain from a deadly disease, such as cancer and angina pectoris
- Chronic pain from a nondeadly disease, such as arthritis
- Chronic pain from unknown causes (psychogenic: "It's all in your head.") such as headaches and some low back pain
- Chronic pain from neurological disorders such as phantom limb and tic douloureux
- Chronic pain caused by prolonged, intermittent diagnostic and treatment procedures as in cases of leukemia and severe burns

This last type of chronic pain might be called iatrogenic. The word means "physician caused" and until fairly recently was seldom heard outside medical circles; but malpractice suits are making it more widely known among lawyers and their clients. Iatrogenic chronic pain is not something resulting from carelessness or ignorance, but incidental to medical procedures. Doctors seem to disregard this type of suffering not indifferently, but in a curious, fatalistic way as if patients should be grateful that every effort is being made to save their lives.

If in the treatment process a patient is burned by radiation, or loses half his face from mutilating surgery, or is so stressed by kidney dialysis that he talks about killing himself, some physicians and clinical scientists brutally confront the patient with the alternative—

death. These physicians and scientists have not yet considered the alternatives, that patients could be better prepared psychologically to cope with pain inherent in certain types of prolonged treatment, that psychotherapists could be brought into the situation to help the patient, even to predict how well a patient will survive long-term iatrogenic chronic pain, and that pain specialists could help alleviate it. When physicians and clinical scientists change their attitudes about this type of pain, it will take its place in medical history as one of medicine's unnecessary horrors.

The self-conscious efforts of physicians to disregard the pain they cause, unable in some instances to control their sense of helpless guilt, account to an extent for their failure to warn patients of the prolonged pain they will experience from corrective surgery. A surgeon who persuaded an elderly woman to have a knee operation to alleviate arthritic pain neglected to tell her that the pain following the operation would be worse than that before, but that eventually she would feel far less pain. The woman was so enraged by the severe pain following surgery and the almost unendurable physical therapy that, after the first session, she kicked the therapist in the shins, a kick any amateur psychologist would tell you was really intended for the surgeon.

Sigmund Freud's experience in being treated for cancer of the mouth grimly illustrates iatrongenic chronic pain. In February 1923, Freud discovered a thick, white patch on his palate, leucoplakia commonly found in the mouths of heavy smokers, as Freud certainly was. At an outpatient clinic in Vienna, Freud's doctor removed the leucoplakia under local anesthetic.

As Dr. Ernest Jones recounts in *The Life and Work of Sigmund Freud*, when Freud's daughter, Anna, went to get her father at the clinic, she found him sitting alone in the outer clinic room, his clothes covered with blood. The operation "had not gone as expected." Too weak to walk, Freud was put on a cot in a small room occupied by a cretinous dwarf. During the night, Freud's incision hemorrhaged. He was unable to speak or call out. And the bell for the nurse didn't work. The dwarf saved Freud's life by going for help.

That operation ominously foreshadowed what was to follow during the next sixteen years. The leucoplakia was cancerous. More and more tissue was removed, then the upper jaw and palate, major surgery performed under local anesthesia. His mouth was fitted with a cumbersome mechanical jaw he called "the monster." Though it made speaking and eating almost impossible, impaired his hearing, and constantly irritated the tissues of his mouth, he had to wear the monstrous prosthesis in order to speak at all. His only source of income was from treating patients. Unless he could talk to them, he would have no patients.

While enduring the succession of operations and re-fittings of the mechanical jaw, Freud continued to treat patients and write books and articles in an effort to get his theories accepted by the medical profession. Dr. Jones says in his biography that, whatever his distress, Freud never showed a sign of irritability or annoyance. After thirty-three operations in sixteen years, a refugee from the Nazis (Hitler acknowledged him by burning his books), Freud, exhausted, suffering indescribable pain, died in London.

The unmitigated suffering Freud endured at the well-intentioned hands of his medical colleagues, had it been inflicted on him in a concentration camp, would have been cited as an example of Nazi brutality. As it was, the sincerity of his physicians in trying to save his life in some way absolved them from responsibility for mitigating the suffering they caused.

Dr. Richard Sternbach, a psychologist at Scripps Clinic Medical Institutions in California, makes an interesting distinction between acute and chronic pain. In the former, all systems are "up" as the automatic system—the "flight or fight" response—prepares the body for coping with the stress of acute illness or an injury. In chronic pain, all systems are "down," the acute pain pattern diminishing, gradually replaced by loss of sleep, appetite, libido, and interest.

Dr. Sternbach charts the contrast in this way:

Acute (Autonomic changes)	Chronic (Vegetative)
↑ Heart rate	↓ Sleep
↑ Sweat	↓ Appetite
↑ Blood pressure	↓ Interests
↑ Muscular tension	↓ Libido

According to Dr. C. Norman Shealy, neurosurgeon and director of the Pain and Health Rehabilitation Center in La Crosse, Wisconsin, the typical chronic pain patient at his center is middle-aged and the survivor of four unsuccessful operations on his back. His pain is from 4 to 10 years' duration. Before seeking help at the center, he has spent as much as $75,000 for medical bills. Almost two-thirds of these patients have chronic low back pain. The typical patient, when he or she arrives at the center for treatment, is addicted to narcotic drugs or tranquilizers and sedatives. Of 24 patients entering Dr. Shealy's clinic at the same time, "only one will be taking nothing stronger than aspirin. When they come in they are clinging desperately to the drugs upon which they have become dependent. Their make-up kits and briefcases are filled with drugs. . . . Conventional physicians are helpless with patients like these. In the treatment of chronic pain the American medical profession is at its weakest."[1]

In medical practice, anything chronic is a "downer." The very word *chronic* evokes an image of morose passivity. Medical school faculty members teach medicine as if their students would spend full time in emergency rooms, training them for crisis, dramatic and spectacular medicine, drug formulas for controlling acute pain, and the flashy diagnosis of obscure disorders. This is seen even in the way medical students are "recruited" for medical specialties. Surgeons, hematologists, dermatologists, obstetricians, cardiologists, every specialist who teaches at medical schools picks out the dramatic aspects, intriguing cases, and spectacular cures of his or her specialty. As one physician admitted, if they presented their specialties the way they are in daily practice year in and year out, some specialties would die out for lack of recruits. And the student, never forgetting what lured him into medical practice, the promise of high drama and cures, never quite recovers from the shock of reality, discovering that in medical practice in America 50 percent of physicians are closet geriatricians.

The attitude of most physicians toward chronic pain is similar to that displayed by some Japanese soldiers during World War II. The incident, told to me years later by a survivor of a Japanese prisoner of war camp, occurred as a group of captured American soldiers, escorted by Japanese guards, were marching through a jungle to a Japanese prison camp. When occasionally an American soldier collapsed from the torrid heat, his comrades picked him up and carried him. The heat also felled an occasional Japanese guard. When that happened, his comrades solicitously doused him with buckets of water. But, if the fallen guard did not revive, his enraged comrades beat him furiously with the empty buckets and abandoned him in the jungle.

If people claim they hurt but show none of the visible signs of suffering, doctors suspect them of being neurotic and either give them drugs to reduce anxiety or refer them to another doctor. There is, however, another type of patient the doctor believes, but cannot help, the patient with tic douloureux, considered in its advanced stages one of the most excruciating of all forms of physical suffering.

The French surgeon René Leriche gives an account of a man who came to him complaining of occasional attacks of severe pain in the jaw. Upon examining the jaw, Dr. Leriche could not find an identifiable reason for the pain. But the attacks not only became more frequent but spread over the man's face. His entire life became dominated by fear of triggering an attack of the pain. The slightest movement of his lips, a twitch of a facial muscle provoked a violent attack. Alternating between dread and pain, he dared not brush his teeth or shave, even feared to speak. Gradually, he withdrew from professional and family life. Utterly debased by pain and fear, he spent his days and nights in despair like an entrapped animal.

In each of us there is a point at which we perceive pain, a threshold that rises and falls in response to myriad influences. Whether we are born with the threshold at a certain level or whether that level is determined by training and circumstances is not known. For most of us, the threshold is of no great significance. What is important to us and to physicians is that it changes and pain control should be adjusted to it.

In laboratory studies of analgesics, investigators measure the length of time it takes a subject, human or animal, to perceive pain after being given the analgesic. But laboratory tests of a drug's efficacy in preventing the perception of pain cannot duplicate the actual experience of pain in people who are sick or injured, beset by anxiety and fear, and who, unlike the subjects taking part in laboratory experiments, cannot signal an attendant to turn off the pain.

Our response to pain depends on how we perceive and interpret it. Our first reaction to sudden, intense pain from a minor injury is apt to be anger, especially if the injury results from our own or someone else's carelessness. After a shocked elderly lady called the telephone company to complain about the obscene language a lineman working on the pole in her backyard had been shouting at his teammate, a supervisor called the lineman and asked him to explain what happened. "Well," the lineman said, "Joe was up the pole and I was down below and he drops the hammer on my head and I says to him, 'Joe, you should be more careful.'"

The pain of minor cuts, broken bones, sprains, or toothaches, intense as it may be, rarely arouses profound anxiety and depression. This type of acute, temporary pain is a survival tool, a teacher, a disciplinarian. The brain interprets the sensation as transitory, not in the least life-threatening. "This will bother you for a week or two," the doctor says, putting a fence around the pain, making it easier to tolerate. Dentists who have control switches for patients to shut off the drill if pain is too much find that even their most anxious patients, once they know they can control the pain, tolerate it much longer than they did before they could throw the switch.

People who understand that pain is inherent in the healing process are less anxious after surgery, though their pain may be intense. A woman giving birth to a baby she wants very much responds to the pain of childbirth quite differently from a woman whose baby was sired by a rapist. In "natural childbirth," the woman's pain perception is conditioned by psychological preparation for "riding out the labor pains," learning appropriate breathing exercises for the peaks and valleys of pain and learning how to relax the rest of the body without interfering with the muscles that must push out the baby. Given a sense of control, women ameliorate their pain perception.

Where our ancestors came from has a lot to do with how we experience and interpret pain. Dr. Irving K. Zola of Brandeis University's Department of Sociology, in his studies of ethnic influences on people's reactions to pain, found that people of Irish and Italian origins responded to pain in quite different ways. The Irish tended to be stoical and precise about the location of the pain. "Right here, doctor." Italians, on the other hand, described their pain in a general, melodramatic way. "It hurts all over.'" In another study, this one of hospitalized Jews, investigators observed that Jewish patients were less concerned about pain itself than about the effect their illness would have on their future and their families.

It would be a mistake to interpret half-empty churches as a sign that religion no longer profoundly influences our moral and emotional responses. The question, "Why me?" is one that every hospital social worker has probably heard hundreds of times. What it implies is: "Why should I, a good, kind, law-abiding person be afflicted by such suffering? What have I done to deserve it?"

Theologians and philosophers for centuries have grappled with the mystery and meaning of pain and suffering. Every major religion considers the matter from its unique point of view and sets forth precepts as guidance for its followers. Even though we might not know precisely what those concepts are, their essence is absorbed from attitudes of parents in the home, from religious services in church or temple. What we may think is an automatic response to pain and suffering most likely has been conditioned in us by the religious beliefs of our ancestors.

Let's consider some of these concepts, starting with Judaism, the most ancient of the major modern religions. There is scarcely a facet of pain and suffering that is not covered by rabbinical law. Though the Jewish faith does not draw a sharp line between ill health and pain, the religious laws address the subject of pain directly. Very early in their religious history, the Jews faced the conflict between accepting suffering as "divine visitation" and the obligation to mitigate suffering through medical intervention. Though much debated by Jewish scholars, the concept that has prevailed is that man "must not rely on miracles or Providence only, but must himself do whatever he can to maintain his life and health."

The Jewish attitude toward pain is that, whether or not it is an instrument of divine punishment, "it is clearly a curse." Judaism attributes no virtue to bodily suffering, a condition not to be sought, but to be avoided. Jewish religious law is specific about many aspects of pain to be ameliorated, especially the pains of childbirth and the suffering of the dying. Even the suffering of animals draws rabbinical attention.

Buddhism, established in the sixth century B.C., considers pain and suffering the "first Noble Truth." Their value is in moving the sufferer to search for and understand their cause. Though Buddhism does not deny the reality of the body's experience of pain or pleasure, it teaches that the body cannot act or react without involving the mind. If the mind is serene, there is no cycle of action and reaction, of suffering begetting suffering. Life is a mind-body combination. Through study and meditation, this mind-body can be brought into a state of equilibrium in which the perception of suffering is diffused.

Since the 1960s, precepts of Buddhism have been widely adopted by young American men and women, and psychotherapists in pain management recommend meditation as a method of therapy.

Between Christians and Jews, considering their common roots in the Bible, there is a striking divergence in views on pain. Christians spiritualize it in the name of Christ, citing His suffering on the cross as the model for all suffering. From the very beginning of Christianity, its followers have preached the virtues of suffering: redemption, expiation, retribution. The many Christian sects interpret pain and suffering in their own ways, but underlying them all is the concept that pain and suffering are visited upon us as punishment for sins, not merely our own personal sins, but the sins of others, too. Women, for instance, were expected to endure the pain of childbirth in expiation of the sin of Eve.

Some Christian theologians and members of the laity have been hard pressed to reconcile the concept of a loving God with One who inflicts unspeakable suffering on those He loves. An interpretation is that God uses suffering as a way of reminding man of His existence, drawing him back when man strays from Him. Another is that it is a test of faith. In medieval times, when not much could be done to mitigate physical suffering, the Catholic Church urged the faithful to offer up their sufferings to God. Today the Catholic Church is ambivalent about pain and suffering. But among many young

Catholic theologians, pain is no longer considered a "Christian good."

The Islamic religion, founded in the sixth century a.d., teaches that pain and suffering, like all other happenings, are manifestations of Allah's will, to be accepted without questioning the wisdom and justice of that will, although it is believed that misfortunes may be caused by an individual's own sin. Patience and fortitude, however, are abundantly rewarded by God and pain and misfortune can be God's way of absolving sins. In contrast to the Christian religion with its emphasis strongly on the suffering of Christ, the Koran touches only briefly on the sufferings of Muhammad. Islamic teachings, rather than addressing pain and suffering as entities, emphasize *sabr:* forbearance, silence and steadfastness under the blows of fate, refraining from complaints, and "welcoming illness as if it were health."

To the Christian Scientist, pain is not a physical thing. The Christian Science concept is that pain is in the mind. God Himself does not suffer pain. What is real is God-like or God-expressed and, in that sense, pain is not real. Christian Science teaches that from God's point of view, pain is illegitimate and disputes His universal harmony. The basis of Christian Science healing is a strong belief in the presence and power of God, evoked through prayer. When God changes one's perspective on pain, it is alleviated.[2]

Even people who might classify themselves as being without religious beliefs have had their attitudes toward pain and suffering influenced by precepts they may never have heard uttered, but which come down to them from one generation to another in teachings of moral and social behavior. Many of these teachings account for the unnamed dread, sense of guilt, and depression of most pain sufferers.

Some who put a perverted value on suffering are reluctant to let it go. When pain specialists sense they are dealing with such a person, they often decide to alleviate the pain only to a certain extent, enough so the person can live a reasonably full life, but not enough to create such a void that the person cannot adjust to it. There have been instances of people committing suicide after losing the "beloved symptom."

Anyone who suffers constant pain for at least six months is bound to develop what psychologists call patterns of pain behavior, individual ways of coping with the stress. A few decades ago, the caricature of an old man was one bent over with one hand pressing the small of his back. Some people, restrained by the fear of hurting, continue to limp even though a sprain is cured and the pain gone. Such outward manifestations are easy to spot. More difficult is assessing psychological adjustments to continuous pain. Yet these reactions often block successful rehabilitation and are used for financial gains, sympathy, and privileged status in the household.

A fairly common situation in nursing homes is the mask of serenity some elderly women put on for nurses and aides. But when sons or daughters visit, there are complaints about the food, the nursing care, the other residents, and persistent pain for which they receive "no relief whatsoever." Family members discover that their mother has never mentioned her pain to the staff, usually for fear of antagonizing them.

Some elderly people who have had mild strokes realize that their ability to concentrate and remember has deteriorated and are pathetically ashamed. Seeking ways of avoiding the stigma of senility, they invent pain as the reason they can no longer sit for hours at a bridge table or keep up with church activities.

People who have the best chance for transcending pain are those with a compelling purpose. To them pain is an enemy to be conquered. Alain Colas and John F. Kennedy proved this, refusing to allow pain to deter them.

Alain Colas, the French solo navigator, set his sights on winning the 1976 Transat, the transatlantic, east-west solo sailboat race, and beating his rival, Eric Tabarly, another famous French solo navigator. Colas, who had sailed more than 120,000 miles of the Atlantic and Pacific oceans and survived about every kind of a disaster that can plague a man alone in a sailboat on the open sea in all weathers, had designed a marvel of an electronic sailing boat for the 1976 Transat. The boat builders were enthusiastic. Colas was stimulating the interest of possible financial backers.

Then, while dropping anchor in a sailboat in a French harbor, Colas stepped over the streaking anchor rope. It looped and caught his foot above the ankle, instantly gouging the flesh and splintering the bone. Swiftly, Colas cut the rope. His foot hung by threads.

Skillful French surgeons at the hospital in Nantes operated, trying to save the foot; but after three months, doubtful that Colas could endure the excruciating pain any longer, they advised that the foot be amputated.

But Alain Colas was determined to sail his fabulous electronic sailboat in the Transat and beat Eric Tabarly. He would not allow his foot to be amputated. His hospital room became his office from which he supervised the building of the boat. To keep a clear head for consultations with the boat builders, he cut down on pain medication. Over the phone he projected the impression of a vital, confident man, persuading possible financial backers and doubtful investors that he would be fit to sail his boat alone across the Atlantic and win.

To get in the best possible physical shape for the series of operations, grafting flesh from one leg to the other, Colas followed a schedule of exercises despite incredible pain. Six months after his accident, Colas left the hospital in Nantes, walking with canes, each step agony. He then began retraining as an athlete, preparing himself for the rigors of the race. In public, closely observed for a sign of weakness, he controlled any expression of pain as he put his weight on the reconstructed foot and slowly walked the docks.

He was advised against participating in the Transat. Nothing could stop him. On June 5, 1976, he sailed out of Plymouth Harbor in England, slightly behind his rival, Tabarly. One hundred twenty-six sailboats, each with a crew of one, headed across the Atlantic for Newport, Rhode Island, and America's Bicentennial celebration. The gales were the worst in years. Only 41 boats finished, some turned back, many were lost at sea.

On July 2, Tabarly sailed into Newport Harbor, the winner. Behind him, in second place, Alain Colas. In New York Harbor, July 4, his own tall-masted boat joined the picturesque "tall ships" that had sailed from countries throughout the world to America to honor its 200th birthday. More important than a trophy Colas could put on his mantelpiece was the foot he could put on the deck.

Dr. Janet Travell, personal physician to John F. Kennedy while he was president, is convinced that those who are too busy to be overwhelmed by pain are the most likely to transcend it. Her own experience with pain she describes in the opening paragraph of her autobiography, *Office Hours: Day and Night*: ". . . I lay flat on my back with my neck held rigid in a steel collar. Chin braced high, I slept in the collar, ate in the collar, and in fact, wore it twenty-four hours a day."

Dr. Travell, in her fifties at the time, had ruptured a disk in her neck while trying to close a car door. A week after the injury, immobilized at home in New York City, she received a phone call from Dr. Ephraim Shoor asking her to see one of his patients who was suffering from a complicated back problem. When Dr. Travell explained her own plight, Dr. Shoor told her this young man was a very special person, Jack Kennedy from Massachusetts, on leave from the United States Senate. The young senator was in a New York hospital for a checkup after a spine fusion about six months before. The spinal operation had not corrected the back problem.

A month later, in May 1955, Senator Kennedy went to Dr. Travell's office. "At our first meeting," she says in her book, "the thin young Senator on crutches could barely navigate the few steps down from the sidewalk into my ground-floor office. Left-sided pain in his back and leg made it almost impossible for him to bear weight on that foot, and a stiff right knee since a football injury in his youth made it difficult for him to step up or down with his weight on the right foot, because that required bending the right knee."

During that office visit, while sitting in Dr. Travell's rocking chair, Kennedy commented on its comfort. When she began his treatment in the hospital, she had the rocking chair taken apart so it would fit in her car and took it to the hospital where it was reassembled and kept in Kennedy's room. Before the end of 1955, he was in Palm Beach writing *Profiles in Courage,* and sitting at the table opposite him was Dr. Travell.

During the years Kennedy's time and energy had been eroded by his constant fight with pain, he had, as Dr. Travell says, "learned the discipline of disability and he had to relearn the freedom of mobility. In Florida that

December, he recovered his trust in his health. He could swim in the ocean again. When he had an ache in his back, he understood that mechanical causes contributed to it and that they could be corrected. The prospect of chronic ill health need not hamper him in his high purpose."

In 1961, Dr. Travell went to the White House with President Kennedy as his personal physician. Indoctrinated by her in the importance of preventing back pain, he asked her to apply her knowledge of proper seating and sitting to the design of chairs for him in the Executive Office, the Cabinet room, on his private and official boats, his helicopters, his official plane, in the bubble-top presidential limousine, and, of course, in his famous rocking chair.

At the Royal Victorian Hospital at McGill University in Montreal, Dr. Ronald Melzack, professor of psychology, and his associates have compiled a list of more than 100 words that patients in the pain clinic check to describe the nature of their pain and its varying intensity. Some of the words on the list are: lancinating, excruciating, crushing, prickling, drilling, throbbing, pulsing. The more intense the pain, the more words patients chose to describe it. The most severe pains are those from certain types of cancer, sciatica, and phantom limb. By focusing on 20 key words from the master list of more than 100, Dr. Melzak works out a pain-rating index used as a basis for treatment.

These are ready-made words pain patients check off to describe how they perceive their pain. But when a professional writer puts words together to describe his sensations, we discover the person behind the patient and the essence of the pain sensation. In 1924, in northern France, a train jumped the tracks in a tunnel and seconds later a train coming from the opposite direction plowed into it. Of the survivors, most were horribly injured, but one man survived with his only injury a broken shinbone. He was Walter Duranty, British journalist, who at the time was foreign correspondent for the *New York Times*.

In a French hospital, doctors tried to save his foot, but those were the days before antibiotics and sophisticated surgery. In his book, *I Write As I Please*, Duranty says, "My leg was a river of pain in which I lay drowning, wave after wave of pain, ninety every minute, one for each hurried heartbeat. . . . How well I knew that Socrates was right, that no pleasure, not even love's orgasm, can compare in joy and splendor with release from pain."

When the nurse left a box of morphine tablets on his bedside table, Duranty suspected she was encouraging him to commit suicide, partly to free him from agony and partly to get rid of a patient who required much care. He resisted the escape, though, as he says, "To swallow one by one the bitter tablets, slowly, in delicious anticipation; the pain beats would grow less sharp, less frequent, be lulled soon to nothing and their victim would float away on rosy clouds of peace and happiness —to peace and death. I did not want to die so I let the morphine alone."

Despite heroic efforts by the physicians and Duranty to save the foot, gangrene set in. The foot was amputated. A dapper, vain little man, Duranty was deeply depressed by his changed self-image. His friend, William Bolitho, also a British journalist, using age-old principles of psychotherapy, took him to a Paris café and, over numerous brandies, gave him a talk about the advantages of disadvantages. Any fool, Bolitho said, can capitalize his gains, but it takes brains to profit from losses. Among the horde of fiercely competitive foreign correspondents swarming in Paris at the time, a journalist needed more than intelligent questions to single him out with important officials and diplomats, the sources of exclusive interviews and stories. A journalist needed some distinguishing physical characteristic. Duranty's limp would mark him out. Bolitho's prophesy was fulfilled. Duranty won a coveted assignment to Russia and became famous as the *New York Times* "Man in Moscow."

Among those who develop the highest pain thresholds are battered children and professional football players. Both groups are motivated by the drive for survival, the children having learned that screams of pain bring on more punishment, the football players controlling their expressions of pain to stay in the game and keep their jobs.

Watching football games on television, you wince at the impact of those giants, yet they get up and walk off casually. It's only the next day, in newspaper accounts, that you find out what happened to them and marvel at human endurance. Football has become a "blood sport," according to psychiatrist Dr. Arnold J. Mandell, whose professional assignment with the San Diego Chargers to figure out their psychological problems nearly wrecked him.

His account of this experience in his book *The Nightmare Season* is a back-door view of professional football. "Big men hurt each other much more," he says. At halftime in the locker room, trainers, and physicians work frantically to patch up the players. "Broken ribs were being X-rayed; hyperextended knees were being taped, fingers splinted, a swollen knee taped; large violaceous bruises were being poked for deeper hurts."

The trainers, practicing what Dr. Mandell calls "a combination of orthopedics and witchcraft," are on the lookout for complainers or those whose thresholds for physical punishment are low. "Pain and depression after games gets worse with each succeeding year. To labor up past baseline to the heights of confidence and energy is a long painful weekly trek. Most of the older players can't do it without help. The existential hate required to win burns out in one's late twenties unless something agitates the centers of rage and aggression in the brain—personal vendettas, fear of starvation, tirades by head coaches, metaphysical trips, alcohol withdrawal, stimulants or antidepressants. Post-game depression magnifies the physical agonies of the bruises, pulled muscles, cracked ribs, trick knees, plantar fascial strain, hematomas, hip pointers, low back pain, cervical strains. It causes impotence, irritability, insomnia, self-torture." Dr. Mandell's endurance fell far short of that of his "patients"—the nightmare experience nearly ruined his career.

Not all players can take the punishment. Paul Laaveg, one of the Washington Redskin's most talented offensive linemen, told Leonard Shapiro of the *Washington Post,* in August 1977, "I have the neck of an old man. I'm tired of treatments and I'm tired of the pain, so I'm quitting." Laaveg, 29 years old, had developed a combination of arthritis, rheumatism, and spurs in the neck. "It wakes you up in the middle of the night," he told Shapiro. "Your arms go to sleep depending on what side you sleep on and I wake up half the time with headaches." In the Houston game, he felt he was losing the feeling in his right arm. "It was something that had been coming on all during the season and I just couldn't take it any more."

But there are dozens waiting to step into the jerseys of players who have had enough. A young college football player who had already developed arthritis told sports writer Mark Asher of the *Washington Post*, "A knee isn't life or death. If it gets stiff when I'm 30, it gets stiff. I knew I was taking that chance when I was 17.

"'You want to play. . . . You don't think about getting old when you're 20. You don't think about how you're going to feel when you're 50. When you think about playing hurt, you think about the present. Athletes have tremendous egos. College athletics is entertainment; like show business, the game must go on. You get lost in a time warp. You think about now; tomorrow seems an eternity away." Present pain and possible future disability are "the price of athletics, the price of winning. The world doesn't need any more losers. . . . You start playing because it's fun. You get your name in the paper, people clap and it makes your parents proud. It goes on through high school, only the stakes are higher. Now it's a business. I knew if I played well in high school I'd get a scholarship. The only difference between college and the pros is $20,000."

The people who get shortest shrift from pain specialists are those who collect disability payments for chronic low back pain. Some pain clinics refuse to accept patients who receive workmen's compensation or who are involved in suits over personal injuries. Neurosurgeons are especially leery of such patients. Sometimes persuaded by pleading, convinced the person really wants to be cured, surgeons have operated only to be confronted a few months later with: "It still hurts, doctor." Does it? The surgeon has no way of knowing.

"What we need," says Dr. James Peter Murphy, neurosurgeon in Bethesda, Maryland, "is some way of measuring pain, not the subjective responses in an experimental setting where the subject knows he can stop the experiment when the pain gets to a certain point, but a measurement that indicates physiological changes caused by pain. This is an area where research money could be well spent and would repay the cost a thousand fold."

At New York University Medical Center, Dr. B. Berthold Wolff and his associates are studying ways of doing just that, developing techniques for measuring pain that could be the basis for evaluating the degree of disability associated with pain. A further aim of these studies is to use the findings of pain and disability measurement tests to predict the likely outcome of pain management treatments, always the most difficult kind of evaluation. Beneficiaries of such studies will be workers locked into the "disability process," and state rehabilitation specialists trying to help them escape.

The *disability process* is a term that includes psychosocial factors that turn comparatively mild physical disabilities into a way of life. Dr. William R. Halliday, medical director of the state of Washington's Department of Social and Health Services, says, "Chronic pain is the presenting complaint in about 98 percent of persons enmeshed in the *disability process*. Of those, 85 percent have chronic low back pain as their chief complaint."

Washington State's workers' compensation program in 1977 was dealing with a third generation of "industrial back" cases, a phenomenon that started in the days when lumberjacks were clearing the forests throughout the state. "Working in the woods," Dr. Halliday explains, "Grandad's back wore out by the time he was 60, and since the straw that broke his back was a minor injury, 'The State' gave him a pension until he died at 88. By the time his sons came along, there was a local tradition of 'retiring on the State' at about age 50—maybe 45 if you lived out in the woods and raised a few chickens. Now we are dealing with whole families of workers in their late 20's, some of whom already have had a couple of back operations, though there were no standard indications for surgery. And too many of those men never work again. That kind of person can and does cost our workers' compensation program as much as a paraplegic. As provided by law, we pass these costs along to the other employees and employers in Washington State, and the latter are not backward in passing them along to the consumer, compounding the impact considerably." Washington State's workers' compensation program costs industry and labor more than $100 million a year.

The *disability process* puts a severe strain on doctor-patient relations. The doctor is inappropriately expected to be a vocational expert and to judge whether or not his patient is able to perform certain jobs about which the doctor knows little or nothing besides what his patients tell him. Commonly, he relies on his patient to tell him how much work he can do and, based on that subjective information, makes his recommendations. A doctor who evaluates a disability as being less than the patient says it is may be subjected to retaliation, especially in small communities where, as Sinclair Lewis describes in *Arrowsmith*, small-town persecution of a doctor can be vicious. Dependent as he is on the goodwill of the town's citizens, a doctor, against his better judgment, may become part of the disability racket.

Dr. Halliday says that many of the workers trapped in the "disability process" are "quiet, hopeless individuals, who don't see life as having anything left for them any more. Others are loud and desperate. Most were self-respecting individuals who, before their injuries, were a credit to their communities, families, unions, employers, and themselves. These are the people that our disability prevention program is especially designed to protect from the tragic involutional spiral that we see all too often as these unfortunates fit their lives into a self-defeating pattern of maintaining a privileged status as disabled."

A remarkable minority, too engaged in their affairs and in living to be hampered by disabling pain, is described by Dr. Sternbach in *Pain Patients:*[3] "If they are unable to perform at their former job, they find something else that they can do, sometimes going to school for retraining. If they accept disability compensation, which is rare, it is only for a brief interim period. They seem proud of their independence and ability to overcome their handicaps, but the motivation seems to be the enjoyment of accomplishment rather than the need to prove anything to others."

I encountered a taxi driver who was such a person. A talkative fellow, he was going on about people being too inquisitive. "Like," he said testily, "people always asking me how I lost my arm." Until that moment, I had not noticed that he had no right arm, just empty space beneath the edge of his short-sleeve shirt. "What do you tell them when they ask you that question?" I said, steaming with curiosity. "I tell them it's none of their damn business." Well, no matter. There he was, without a right arm, earning his living driving a taxi.

It's unfair to give pain a totally bad name, not to acknowledge it as our first teacher, training us to live safely with danger, setting alarms warning us of internal disorders. It also teaches good manners. A friend of mine says that the best way to teach a child civility is to give him a cat. If he tortures it, he quickly learns from the cat's claws and teeth, if not kindness, at least respect for another living creature.

Occasionally, someone is born without the ability to perceive pain. At the University of Washington, scientists put together the history of a 25-year-old man who had never felt pain. When he was 10 months old, he bit off the tip of his tongue and didn't utter a sound. Five months later, he severely burned his hands, again without any sign of distress. Throughout his life this unfortunate young man suffered a series of mutilating injuries to which he was oblivious. At 25, he was a deformed cripple.

His case gives us some appreciation of the value of pain, but how many of us would go so far as to venerate it? A few religious fanatics, you might suppose. But a great orthopedic surgeon? Dr. Paul Brand arrived in London after an exhausting transatlantic ocean trip and long train ride from the English coast. He was getting ready for bed, had taken off his shoes, and, as he pulled off a sock, discovered there was no feeling in his heel. To most anyone else this discovery would have meant very little, a momentary numbness. But Dr. Brand was world famous for his restorative surgery on lepers in India. He had convinced himself and his staff at the leprosarium that there was no danger of infection from leprosy after it reached a certain stage. The numbness in his heel terrified him.

In her biography of Dr. Brand, *Ten Fingers for God*, Dorothy Clarke Wilson says, "He rose mechanically, found a pin, sat down again, and pricked the small area below his ankle. He felt no pain. He thrust the pin deeper, until a speck of blood showed. Still he felt nothing. . . . He supposed, like other workers with leprosy, he had always half expected it. . . . In the beginning probably not a day had gone by without the automatic searching of his body for the telltale patch, the numbed area of skin"

All that night he tried to imagine his new life as a leper, an outcast, his medical staff's confidence in their immunity shattered by his disaster. And the forced separation from his family. As night receded, he yielded to hope and in the morning, with clinical objectivity, "with steady fingers he bared the skin below his ankle, jabbed in the point—and yelled."

Blessed was the sensation of pain! He realized that during the long train ride, sitting immobile, he had numbed a nerve. From then on, whenever Dr. Brand cut his finger, turned an ankle, even when he suffered from "agonizing nausea as his whole body reacted in violent self-protection from mushroom poisoning, he was to respond with fervent gratitude, 'Thank God for pain!' "[4]

Out of his own experience, the shock and relief, he became intensely interested in the phenomenon of pain and developed an intriguing theory about its possible origins and purpose, far back in time when multicelled organisms were first developing: Individual cells then had to give up their autonomy and learn to suffer with one another and to cooperate for the survival of the higher more complex organism.

In a more practical way, Dr. Brand applied his understanding of pain to the mystery of the erosion of lepers' hands and feet, commonly thought to be a manifestation of the disease itself. In thousands of operations on lepers' rigid claw hands, Dr. Brand, using the extraordinary surgical techniques he had developed, had restored movement to the hands, but not feeling. It was commonly believed that leprosy itself eventually reduced feet and hands to stubs. But observing the hands of his patients months after their operations, Dr. Brand noticed that cuts, abrasions, and blisters injured the skin and flesh of the insensitive hands, gradually eroding them. Feet were eroded as lepers, walking on bare, numb feet, tore flesh and abraded bones on stony roads and rough mountainsides. Rats, too, took a toll, biting off fingers and toes as unaware lepers slept. Many villagers returning home from the leprosarium were given cats as guardians in the night, living replacements for pain-carrying nerves destroyed by leprosy. Dr. Brand, who has already accomplished wonders in rehabilitating lepers, dreamed of finding a way to restore the sensation of pain.

3 | the Cancer Industry

The multibillion-dollar cancer industry is a triumph for disease terrorists. As loaded emotionally as the word *leprosy* was in biblical times, the word *cancer* conjures up death, mutilation, agonizing pain. The power of the word to raise money is a fund-raising phenomenon. The Congress has awarded billions of public funds to the National Cancer Institute. The American Cancer Society raises each year well over $100 million. Other aggressive national fund-raising cancer agencies include: Cancer Research Institute, Chemotherapy Foundation, Damon Runyon-Walter Winchell Cancer Fund, Leukemia Society of America, National Cancer Cytology Center, National Leukemia Association, United Cancer Institute, and the National Foundation for Cancer Research.

Dr. Robert Hadsell of the National Cancer Institute says there are numberless local agencies, impossible to count or keep track of, many "kookie, quacky" agencies that suddenly appear, raise a bundle of money, and disappear. Then there are healing practitioner groups, sometimes semireligious, whose claims for cures are hard to substantiate. Unregenerate rogues and tricksters rake in from $1 to $2 billion a year for "miracle" cancer cures. Those they defraud are usually the very ill, the very desperate.

51

Some 50 insurance companies gamble conservatively on the chances of people getting cancer by offering special cancer policies, usually for a particular type of cancer. Profits are high for drug companies that sell anticancer drugs, data processing companies producing miles of statistics, and printers who turn out tons of pamphlets, newsletters, fund-raising leaflets and posters, and tomes of reports.

There might be some rationale for this multibillion-dollar industry if cancer were the leading cause of death in America, but each year, 750,000 Americans die from heart diseases compared with 350,000 from cancer. Publicity about cancer, the almost daily press stories about carcinogens in food, air, on farms, and in factories, has raised public awareness of the disease to almost hysterical heights. Cancer is the modern equivalent of leprosy, equally terrifying, socially stigmatizing. Inherent in "cancerophobia" is the dread of prolonged pain and an agonizing death.

Dr. F. J. Ingelfinger, former editor of the *New England Journal of Medicine*, said in an editorial that the American public is convinced that there are two ways of dying, the ordinary and reasonably good way and the bad cancer way:

> American cancerophobia, in brief, is a disease as serious to society as cancer is to the individual—and morally more devastating. For this state of affairs, many are to blame—not only high-pressure advertisers who foment and exploit our cancerophobia, but also well meaning but yet baneful practices of other groups: activist consumer organizations, politicians, and even the American Cancer Society, which points directly accusatory fingers at you if you do not give money to "cure cancer." Among the guilty are the media. Because of our society's disease, any news about cancer, no matter how trivial, is ipso facto sensational. Whether it is the latest tentative suggestion that some agent or condition is oncogenic,

or the most recent molecular definition of the cancer cell's wall, the media treat the tentative indictment as if it were an actual catastrophe, and the minor laboratory discovery is heralded as another "breakthrough" in our "war" against cancer. So the vicious circle spirals upward and outward: cancerophobia elicits sensationalist reporting, which in turn fosters the demonology of cancer.[1]

How justified is the rampant fear and anxiety? In 1937, when the National Cancer Institute was established with a $400,000 annual budget, the disease was not foremost in public or medical consciousness. A standard physiology textbook in medical schools, *The Machinery of the Body*, published in 1937 barely mentions cancer. What has happened since 1937 to transform a $400,000 operation into the multibillion-dollar cancer industry?

The American Cancer Society had been generating fear for years in its fund campaigns. Then came Richard Nixon's "War on Cancer," backed by huge sums from the Congress and flamboyant publicity campaigns that aroused public dread unmatched in medical history. But the public was not to worry—money would buy the cure. Had not money bought a cure for polio? What the public did not understand was that polio was caused by a virus that, once identified, could be prevented by a vaccine. Cancer is quite different, not one, but a hundred variations of a functional disorder, the manufacture of abnormal cells. At the time the National Cancer Institute was established in 1937, when the nature and causes of cancer were largely a mystery, the discovery of a single cure seemed a plausible research goal. By the time the "War on Cancer" was launched in 1974, we knew not much more about the causes of cancer, but we did know that from 80 to 90 percent of cancers were caused in some way by environmental factors, chemicals used in manufacturing processes, in food, polluted air and water, even in some of the medicines commonly used to treat disorders, including cancer itself.

Putting things into perspective, Dr. George J. Cosmides, deputy director, Toxicology Information Program, National Library of Medicine, says, "There are thousands of chemical compounds in our environment, some violently toxic, some apparently innocuous, some slightly toxic, and some we don't know about yet. Our expectations today are so high we forget that man has survived some very unhealthy periods in his evolution. In medieval times he was the victim of his own ignorance, now he's the victim of his own ingenuity."

Since the early 1950s there has been an explosion in chemicals for industrial and medical purposes: drugs, pesticides, food, cosmetics, clothing, dyes, sprays, road construction materials, and cleaners. Some 1,000 new chemical compounds are introduced every year. "It's very difficult in some industries to pin-point exactly which chemical causes cancer," Dr. Cosmides says. "What we have to do is ask the question about risks versus benefits. If a certain chemical essential to a manufacturing process is known to cause cancer, are we willing to close down a plant of thousands of workers? Some towns depend for their existence on one plant.

"Once workers know what the risk is, they, and management, can take steps to mitigate the danger. In physically dangerous work, like construction, the worker has some control; he can predict, avoid, or minimize accidents, but the worker who experiences slow, insidious, irreversible damage from chemicals is helpless. Of course, we must remember that chemicals are selective. Not everyone in a plant develops cancer, nor does cancer afflict everyone in the population."

Cancer rates, despite Herculean efforts by scientists to find the causes of it, and by the American Cancer

Society to educate the public about the importance of early diagnosis, have scarcely changed in the past twenty-five years. The prospect of controlling carcinogens in industry is something not even Hercules himself could do. It becomes more and more evident that the individual can do more to prevent the disease than science.

Is there such a thing as a "cancer type" of person? Dr. John Heller, former director of the National Cancer Institute, gave his version of the cancer type at a meeting of a nonprofessional group. After the meeting, a woman from the audience accosted him and said, indignantly, "Dr. Heller, my sister is not like that at all. She's a *lovely person*." Dr. Heller gave no more public profiles of cancer personality types.

But Dr. Lawrence LeShan, a New York City research psychotherapist, is less reticent. In his book, *You Can Fight for Your Life*, he says that in the course of his research with more than 500 cancer patients, he found that they had a "bottled-up" quality to their emotional lives, that they lacked ways of expressing their emotional energies. Talking with cancer patients, he found that many of them had developed the disease after the death of someone very close to them or following the loss of a job that had been the focus of their lives. They fitted a pattern, that of people who directed their energies on one person or on a career and never developed inner resources that might have sustained them in their loss.

Not everyone is psychologically or emotionally predisposed to cancer. Genetic factors are involved and sometimes the onslaught is inexplicable, as in the case of a concert violinist who, at the age of 40, at the height of his musical career, was told he had lymphosarcoma and would not live for more than six months. Taking matters into his own hands, convinced he had nothing to lose, he went to an obscure clinic in the California desert. Run by a religious group, the clinic combined faith healing with a rigorous diet. For the first month, the violinist was on a liquid diet, then on a diet that allowed no meat, whole milk, sugar, processed foods, or artificial flavorings.

Four months later, he returned home. Six months later, still maintaining the diet, he was examined by doctors who found no trace of cancer. For ten years, in robust health, he taught at Loma Linda University and gave concerts throughout the United States and Europe. At 53, lulled by the complete remission of cancer and harassed by the difficulties of keeping on the diet while traveling, he gave up the stringent diet.

Within months, small tumors developed on his legs. For a while he was given radiotherapy, but when he refused further treatment because of the severe skin burns and pain, the doctors switched to chemotherapy. On a concert tour in Europe, because of an error in translating dosages from one language to another, he received an overdose of the anti-cancer drug. Flown back to the United States in grave condition, his life was prolonged by the amputation of his leg. He continued to give concerts, but gradually the anti-cancer drugs so sensitized his hands he could not play the violin, could not even bear to have his nails clipped. When he realized that to be alive at all meant to play the violin, he regained his virtuosity by diligent practice. Shortly before he died, eighteen years after he had been told he had six months to live, he gave his final concert.

In the space of only a few decades, a mystique of fear and superstition, heavily overlaid with guilt rooted in religious concepts, has enveloped cancer. Some of the elements of this mystique were discussed by Kathryn

Himmelsbach, chief of the Cancer Social Work Section of the National Institutes of Health Clinical Center, the nation's largest research hospital. "The verdict of cancer means death. That's the first reaction, the loaded gun held by a killer. Panic and fear set in. Then, though the gun is kept pointed at the victim, it doesn't go off, merely threatens, and the victim goes through a whole kaleidoscope of emotions. Anger at fate for being singled out. Fear of a future that is doomed but not in a predictable time. There's the fear of pain everyone associates with cancer. And the possible disfigurement from surgery, especially if it is around the face, the jaw, the nose, the cheeks. Or loss of arms or legs. Besides the threat to the bodily integrity, the self-image, there is the fear of being dependent for survival, for care, for everything. Or there may be just the opposite reaction, a complete yielding to dependency, putting the full weight on a spouse and children."

While the person who knows he has cancer is being emotionally battered by his own personal fears and anxieties, those closest to him, his immediate family and close relatives, are coping with their own fears. "Even though hundreds of millions of dollars have been spent on educating the public about cancer," Mrs. Himmelsbach said, "there is widespread belief that it's contagious. Wives are afraid of getting their husband's cancer if they sleep together, neighbors avoid the cancer victim. Even in business, fellow workers make a person with cancer feel subtly ostracized. Having cancer puts people in a kind of apartheid situation. This is the heartbreak that is so hard for cancer patients to endure."

From patients at the clinical center, Mrs. Himmelsbach has heard incredible stories of rejection and even of hostile discrimination against them in their communities. "People who have cancer need so much to have someone who is close to them, who accepts them in spite of physical changes that may occur from treatment methods, surgery and chemotherapy. And who accepts them with the pain that so many cancer patients endure, especially in the final stages of certain types of cancer. They need emotional support from their families, their friends, their clergymen."

And their physicians. "Cancer pain," says Dr. John J. Bonica, "is often improperly treated by physicians and other health professionals. Because it has been neglected by oncologists, investigators, and medical teachers, we don't know enough about its mechanisms and physiopathology and other aspects in order to control it properly."

Much of the information we do have, Dr. Bonica says, is improperly or inadequately applied. "Medical students, physicians, and other health professionals are not instructed in the techniques of managing cancer pain. And practitioners get little help from medical literature on developing long-term cancer pain control. In view of its importance, it is especially surprising that there is an obvious lack of interest in medical literature about the problem, even in oncologic literature. Of the many textbooks on various aspects of cancer, only a few deal with the problem of pain management and then so do in a totally inadequate manner."

Cancer is rarely painful at its onset and pain is by no means present in all cancers. There are no exact figures on its incidence, but one estimate is that it occurs in 15 percent of cancers. In figures, that seems a small percent. In terms of people, it means 435,000 of the 2,900,000 who have cancer. Yet, it is an area of the disease that the major cancer agencies, federal and private, have neglected. The American Cancer Society supported no cancer pain research in 1975, 1976, or 1977. Out of its billion-dollar-a-year budget, the National Cancer Institute spent $600,000 on pain research in 1977.

Dr. Peter Mozden, chief of the Oncology Department of Boston University Hospital, has a higher estimate of cancer patients who have pain—one-fourth to one-third. He advocates that more research be done on drug therapy that changes the perception of pain, especially for those patients in the final stages of the disease. At the time I interviewed him, the strictures on research with heroin, marijuana, and LSD had not been lifted by President Carter, but Dr. Mozden had for years advocated research on those drugs.

"When cancer invades bone, like termites invading wood, there is irritation of nerve endings in the bone, especially vertebrae," Dr. Mozden told me. "Bones sag and collapse and pressure on nerve roots can be excruciating. If breast cancer spreads to the chest bones, the matrix of the bone is destroyed, tiny nerve endings are irritated, and the result is extremely painful." As a tumor of the liver enlarges, the liver lining stretches, causing unbearable pain, and the same is true of distention of the bowel caused by a tumor.

In managing cancer pain, Dr. Mozden considers ameliorating anxiety of first importance. He believes the diagnosis of cancer should be discussed with the patient and the family. The plan for treatment should be explained so that it is not only understood, but the patient's apprehensions allayed.

"Most physicians who make out the daily orders for sedatives or analgesics follow traditional amounts, ordering say 100 mgm of a barbiturate in combination with a pain drug rather than the needed 300 mgm to assure a good night's sleep. There should be no groans on cancer wards because physicians skimp on doses. On the other hand, patients should not be drugged into a stupor. They should be free of pain, but able to function and to converse with family and friends. And if they are in the final stages of their illness, they should be able to make decisions affecting business or household affairs, to leave things in order. Having a patient free of pain, but not anesthetized, not only comforts him, but his family."

Pain management specialists agree that a common fault in cancer pain control is using powerful narcotic analgesics early on for mild to moderate pain, thereby causing premature tolerance. The only alternatives later on if patients need powerful narcotics are to drug them into a stupor or let them suffer. Stewart Alsop, former newspaper columnist, in a television interview some months before his death from leukemia, told about sharing his hospital room with a young man dying of cancer. The man would be given a painkiller, said Alsop, "and about two and a half hours after the drug had been administered, he'd begin to howl like a dog. Or he'd whimper like a dog. And I remember thinking to myself, if he were a dog, what would we do?"

Overdosing a patient with narcotics because a physician thinks the end is near has its own risks, according to Dr. Bonica. Because it is difficult to predict the length of time a person will live, "such false humanitarianism may produce premature respiratory depression, stupefaction, headache, loss of appetite, nausea, vomiting, and emaciation. Since tolerance develops rapidly, the patient may not obtain adequate relief in the later stages, even with massive doses."

In its early stages, cancer pain can be ameliorated by nonnarcotic analgesics and drugs that reduce anxiety. If the cancer itself cannot be controlled by surgery, radiotherapy, or chemotherapy, the treatment of pain becomes a primary consideration, not only to reduce suffering but to maintain the patient's well-being. Keeping him or her in the best possible physical condition, eating and sleeping, anxieties calmed, and morale improved, increases reserves of strength for coping with pain itself. In the later stages of the disease, keeping the patient comfortable is medicine's final obligation.

Intellectually, physicians accept these basic precepts, but, because there is a dearth of explicit, how-to-do-it information, they inadvertently add to the horror stories circulated by distraught members of the families of dying patients. At the time this book was being written in 1977, neither the National Cancer Institute nor the American Cancer Society had set up a task force of physicians, oncologists, and pain specialists to develop protocols for the management of cancer pain. Nor did any of the federally supported cancer research and treatment centers throughout the country have pain specialists as members of their staffs.

One of the two American standard reference books on cancer, Cancer Medicine, edited by Drs. James Holland and Emil Frei, III, scarcely mentions cancer pain management. The other standard reference book, Cancer: Diagnosis, Treatment, and Prognosis by Drs. Lauren V. Ackerman and Juan A. del Regato vividly describes what some patients endure from pain, but gives only passing reference to alleviation. For instance, the authors liken the pain of cancer of the pancreas to that of dogs tearing away the upper part of the abdomen. (Annually, some 20,000 people die of cancer of the pancreas.) Pain onslaughts, the authors say, can be "relieved by sitting up and leaning forward or by lying on the right side with the legs drawn up and bending forward at the hips." Usually more severe at night, the pain makes sleep impossible and, as the disease progresses and the pain intensifies, the patient's distress is complicated by vomiting.

Besides suggesting that patients sit up and lean forward, what advice do the authors of this reference book give physicians in the management of this ravening pain? They cite a study of 91 patients irradiated with cobalt in which ten percent of the patients experienced palliative results considered excellent, "mostly through relief of pain and decrease of jaundice." Small wonder that physicians trying to control cancer pain desperately resort to massive doses of narcotics when their authoritative sources give so little guidance on methodical pain management.

In his book, *Intractable Pain*,[2] a reference book for physicians, British physician Mark Mehta says:

> The *quality of remaining life* should be the sole consideration in a terminal illness which, because it is incurable, can only get worse and, consequently, the main aim of treatment is to make the patient comfortable. Of the many complaints a person in this state may have, continuous pain is by far the worst and its relief merits the highest priority. Table 10.1 lists the many methods available for control of pain, selection depending on many factors, such as age, fitness, personality, temperament, stage of the disease, and probable life expectancy. Only by looking at the entire problem in perspective is it possible to plan a comprehensive schedule, utilizing these different techniques so that at any stage in a long drawn-out malady a fully effective means of securing adequate analgesia is always at hand.

Whether or not American physicians would agree on Dr. Mehta's pain management plan, it provides some idea of the alternatives and it is important for the families of cancer patients to know that there are alternatives. As it is, families are helpless spectators at the

TABLE 10.1 Methods of pain-relief for inoperable cancer

1. GENERAL
    Diet: blood transfusion: general health.
    Reassurance: psychotherapy.
    Comfortable posture—"position of ease."
    Support, e.g. corset or spinal jacket, limb braces or splints.
    Reduced weight bearing and immobilization.
    Elimination of pressure, e.g. drainage of ascites or pleural effusion.
2. CHEMOTHERAPY
    Direct application of cytoxic agents (hollow viscera, e.g. pleura, bladder, extra-dural space).
    Relief of secondary infection by routine drugs, e.g. penicillin.
3. DEEP X-RAY THERAPY
    e.g. relief of nerve compression by bony metastases.
4. GENERAL SURGERY
    Palliative resection.
    Pituitary: adrenal.
    Drainage of abscess, peritoneal fluid, etc.
5. ANALGESIC AND ALLIED DRUGS
    (a) Early stages—mild analgesic and tranquillizers.
    (b) Late—powerful narcotics in large dosage.
6. INHALATIONAL ANALGESIA
    Viz. similar to methods of self-administration used in child birth, e.g. Entonox ($N_2O + O_2$)
7. NERVE BLOCKS (neurolytic agents)
    Individual nerve block.
    Spinal and extra-dural.
    Autonomic block.
    Others, e.g. barbotage, "cold" saline.
8. TEMPERATURE
    e.g. hyper- and hypothermia.
9. "CENTRAL"
    Percutaneous electric cordotomy.
10. NEUROSURGERY
    Neurosurgical procedures.

(Reproduced with permission from *Intractable Pain* by Mark Mehta.)

bedsides of those they love, flinching at every grimace and outcry. Knowing that there are alternatives enables them to discuss with physicians at the outset a plan of long-term pain management.

Another British physician experienced in treating patients with intractable pain is Dr. Robert G. Twycross, consultant physician-in-charge at Sir Michael Sobell House, the Churchill Hospital in Headington, Oxford, England, and at one time research clinical pharmacologist at St. Christopher's Hospice in London. Dr. Twycross is best known in the United States for his studies on narcotic analgesics, especially his work on the relative effectiveness of morphine and heroin in controlling cancer pain. Because American physicians and scientists have been prohibited even from using heroin in research, they have had to base their judgments on the research of Dr. Twycross and others in countries where heroin is considered a useful medication.

In a sense Dr. Twycross has been caught in the middle of the quiet, acrimonious debate between those who oppose legalizing heroin for medicinal use and those who advocate making it available to physicians for controlling terminal cancer pain. The former say Dr. Twycross's studies show that morphine and heroin are equally effective in controlling severe pain; the latter say his studies show unmistakably the superiority of heroin to morphine.

Perhaps the best way to resolve this debate is to let Dr. Twycross speak for himself. In the first place, he says, there is nothing magical about heroin. "It is merely a morphine radical with two molecules of acetic acid tagged on. Called diamorphine in Great Britain, it is widely used there to relieve severe pain in acute situations and also for advanced cancer. When given intravenously, it has an earlier onset of action, is more sedative, and causes less vomiting than morphine. By mouth, because it is metabolized by the gut and by the liver, there is no real difference between orally administered diamorphine and orally administered morphine in terms of analgesic effect and other actions.

"However, about ten percent of patients with advanced cancer and pain require injected medication, either because of intractable vomiting which causes the oral medication to be vomited before it can be fully absorbed, or because the pain is so severe that it fails to respond even to large doses of oral morphine. Such patients may need injected medication every three or four hours. In emaciated patients with little muscle left, a small volume injection is both desirable and humane."

Because heroin is more soluble than morphine, and can be manufactured as freeze-dried pellets rather than supplied in solutions, Dr. Twycross says it is always possible to administer it in a smaller volume than morphine. "Whereas with an injection of diamorphine, the injection need never be more than say one-half milliliter, an equally effective dose of morphine might mean an injection of six, eight, or twelve milliliters ... there is no doubt in my mind that diamorphine is the best and safest of all the potent narcotic analgesics when injections are necessary. There is no doubt that, in the case of patients with advanced cancer, diamorphine is an indispensible medication.

"Legalizing heroin for medicinal use in the United States is one thing. Changing deeply ingrained cultural habits and outlooks is another, calling for sustained effort and a continuing program of education over many years."[3]

President Carter's lifting the restrictions on research with heroin, marijuana, and LSD opens the way for more pain control alternatives. Research already carried out on LSD and marijuana gives us an inkling of the benefits. In the late 1960s, Dr. Walter Pahnke, a psychiatrist formerly at the Maryland Psychiatric Research Center, pioneered in the use of LSD in changing the perception of cancer pain. This "mind opening" drug intensifies sensations whether pleasant or harrowing. It can induce terror, delusions, and deep depression, as experiments carried out by the Central Intelligence Agency on unsuspecting subjects proved when one subject jumped out a window and killed himself. In a supportive setting, LSD can induce quite different reactions.

In a talk Dr. Pahnke gave at the National Institutes of Health in 1969, he described his studies of the effects of LSD on patients dying of cancer. "They were desperate, isolated, in despair, and suffering intense pain," he said. "We prepared them for the LSD experience with intensive psychotherapy. A therapist whom they knew and trusted was with them in the treatment room which we had made as attractive as possible with flowers and soft music. The patients expected something pleasant to happen to them. After taking the LSD, the relief of physical suffering was dramatic. Their anxiety decreased and with it tension. Afterwards, their relations with the staff and their families were noticeably warmer."

Dr. Pahnke's pioneer studies of LSD's beneficent effects on cancer pain were cut short by his death while scuba diving off the coast of Maine in 1971. A few sporadic studies of LSD's effects on pain perception were later carried out, but government strictures on such research discouraged investigators.

At the Sidney Farber Center in Boston, Dr. Stephen Sallan and his associates studied the effects of the active ingredient in marijuana to find out if, as had been rumored, the drug alleviated the almost continuous nausea and vomiting experienced by patients undergoing cancer chemotherapy. In recruiting cancer patients for the experiment, the researchers sought patients in a wide age range. Some older patients demurred, reluctant to try an illicit drug even though it might alleviate their discomfort. Twenty-two patients, ranging in age from 18 to 76, took part in the "double blind" experiment, some patients receiving the marijuana tablet (equal to twelve strong marijuana cigarettes) and others an inert substance (placebo), none of the patients knowing which of the two he or she received.

The results of the study, published in the New England Journal of Medicine,[4] were conclusive: Marijuana not only reduced nausea and vomiting, but enabled some who had lost their appetites to relish food once again. Dr. Sallan told Cristine Russell, science writer on the Washington Star, that after the article appeared in the New England Journal of Medicine, he heard from dozens of physicians, families of patients, and patients themselves, all wanting to know how they could get the drug for medicinal purposes. In each case, reported Cristine Russell, "Sallan has necessarily given the same unsatisfactory answer. Since the drug is illegal, he cannot provide it to those who want to try its medicinal properties." In his replies, Dr. Sallan explained that he was only licensed to use the drug within the Sidney Farber Center under very tightly controlled circumstances, but he hoped that "in the near future, this situation will change." That was in March 1976. In September 1977, the ban on the use of marijuana for research was lifted.

Dr. Sallan's experiences in dealing with federal agencies overseeing marijuana research—the Food and Drug Administration, the Justice Department's Drug Enforcement Administration, and the National Institute on Drug Abuse—were similar to those of other investigators. One scientist, discouraged by the distressing delays and obstructions, concluded, "The hassle just isn't worth it."

A similar conclusion was reached by Dr. Charles Whitfield of Southern Illinois University who told Cristine Russell that his own studies similar to Dr. Sallan's had shown like success, but that he was inclined to give up further studies using the drug because he had "a gut feeling that the government does not want to see anything positive come out of marijuana because politically it is unpopular."

It is understandable that, whatever the possible benefits to cancer or other patients, scientists have approached this type of research gingerly. And there are few hospital administrators who want agents from the Justice Department's Drug Enforcement Administration running all over their hospitals checking on minuscule amounts of marijuana being given to a handful of research patients who, while getting the drug, do not throw up every few minutes. The test of President Carter's reversal of past policy in regard to marijuana, LSD, and heroin will be in how flexibly it is interpreted by law enforcement agencies. Changing their own perceptions may be as difficult for them as it is for chronic pain sufferers to change their ingrained pain behavior.

The public concept of cancer as a death sentence has not yet caught up with advances in treatment. So thoroughly have the "disease terrorists" done their job, that people do not trust the treatment. But the fact is that surgery, radiation, chemotherapy, and immunology are taking cancer out of the "killer" classification and moving it into the chronic disease category.

Chemotherapy, still in an early experimental state, requires delicate adjustments of powerful, toxic chemicals to each patient. The origins of the anti-cancer drugs give some clue to their violent nature. They are an offshoot of research on the deadly mustard gas first used in World War I. It had disastrous effects not only on the enemy—the Germans at that time—but on the British soldiers, who sent the gas cylinders hurtling into the German trenches and shifting winds blew the gas back into the trenches from whence it came.

In World War II, while scientists were experimenting with ways of increasing the devastating effects of mustard gases, several laboratory workers were exposed to the chemical. In treating them, it was discovered that the mustard gases depressed bone marrow and white blood cell counts. Some life-oriented scientists on the project theorized that the chemicals might be used in controlling the growth of malignant cells. Secret clinical trials were conducted on patients with Hodgkin's disease, a cancer of the lymph glands. The results were beneficial, but for military security reasons, no word of this success was released to the medical profession until after the war.[5]

When chemotherapy was first used on cancer patients, many physicians considered the horrendous assault of the chemicals on the body worse than the disease. (Some physicians still feel that way about it.) The chemicals arrest the malignant growth of some cells, but their action cannot be controlled in certain normal cells that have rapid growth and metabolism rates, cells in the bone marrow, gastrointestinal tract, and hair follicles. The result is that patients under chemotherapy treatment experience nausea and vomiting, loss of hair and, in the longer course, rashes, ulcerations in the mouth and gastrointestinal tract, loss of appetite and, understandably, depression.

In the early 1970s, chemotherapy was used largely to control cancer pain. Today, some 50 chemicals are used to control the growth of cancer cells, and the treatment of the disease is still the front-line defense against pain. Yet, even during intensive chemotherapy treatment, besides the offensive side effects, some cancer pain may persist. Powerful analgesics are not always the answer for many patients who lead fairly normal lives, who must be alert enough to run a household of children or work in outside jobs. Thousands of them seek and find psychological and emotional support in groups where they get together to talk about their anxieties and help each other solve personal and family problems that handicap their chances of recovery and affect their perceptions of pain.

Clelia Goodyear, a New York psychotherapist in private practice, has conducted such group sessions with clients, young or middle-aged, able to pay for the therapy, and suffering from some form of malignant cancer. In an interview with Mrs. Goodyear, she told me that one thing she has found in her work with cancer patients is that people who coped successfully with life's problems before becoming ill cope better with the disease than those who managed their lives in a marginal way.

"The patient in pain poses special problems for the therapist," she said. "It's hard for them to give up the role of patient and become an ordinary person who, in the course of his life, handled very well common types of pain like headaches, cramps, and sprains. Once back in the role of the ordinary person, people with cancer can handle more pain than they had thought possible. They accept the fact that 'This is going to hurt' as they do in the dentist's chair. It's remarkable how the ability to tolerate pain can be developed when patients become more active, visit friends, travel, take even short trips that get them out of the circumscribed setting where suffering is exaggerated. As confidence in themselves builds, they get great satisfaction from exerting some control over their condition. Just setting goals for restorative activities helps people manage pain."

Being part of a group, or receiving private counseling, assuages patients, supports them, and prevents total despair. One of Mrs. Goodyear's patients who had returned to the hospital for chemotherapy treatment insisted on taking a few hours' leave from the hospital in order to attend the regular session of his group for a free exchange of talk with those whose own conditions enabled them to understand him better than did his own family.

When a member of a group had a pain flare-up, Mrs. Goodyear helped him or her ferret out any negative influences that might have contributed to the increase in pain intensity. It usually turned out that there is a problem in the family, or exhaustion, or sudden panic. Or it was sometimes due to a change in medication, for, as Mrs. Goodyear said, "Chemotherapy is an artistic mixture of drugs and in its present experimental stage, no one can predict how the mixture will affect a patient."

By mutual support, members of her groups instill in each other the courage to do what they did not believe possible. One timid woman on whom a young hospital resident was practicing taking a blood sample from a groin artery, a painful procedure, was afraid to complain to anyone on the hospital staff. Urged on by her group, she worked up the courage to complain at the hospital. The blood-drawing practice sessions stopped, but then the group had to rally to bolster her morale, for she had been marked out by the hospital staff as a "bad patient."

Helping her clients change their perception of their pain was not so difficult as changing their concepts of themselves as patients. Mrs. Goodyear tried to get them to change their passive attitudes, their sense of helplessness, and to see themselves as medical consumers and relate consumer principles to their medical care. "At present, they, and other cancer patients, are disadvantaged in their care because of the fractionated, diffused approach to cancer treatment, each specialty intent on its own role without considering the patient as a whole person."

Only a few decades ago when "cancer" and "death" were synonyms, to speak of rehabilitating cancer patients seemed a contradiction of terms. But no longer. The American Cancer Society supports rehabilitation programs throughout the country, deploying local trained volunteers to help rehabilitate women who have had breast surgery. Volunteers who have undergone breast removal themselves visit women in hospitals who are adjusting to the traumatic change in their self-image. It's more than a morale-boosting visit, though. The volunteers get down to practicalities, teach the women patients exercises to restore arm muscles and even take them a temporary "falsie" bra. People who have had colostomies, surgery requiring a new opening in the abdominal wall, an operation once mentioned only in whispers, feel less overwhelmed when volunteers who have gone through the same experience instruct them in the special procedures for self-care and help with psychological adjustment. In many communities, American Cancer Society divisions pay certified speech therapists to teach new speaking techniques to those who have had their voice boxes removed.

The chances of successful rehabilitation have improved as more sophisticated surgery reduces disability. Surgeons cut with greater skill, preserving lymph glands, operating in such a way that there are few "big arms" after breast removal. Exercises restore the flexibility of arms after mastectomy. Women can play golf, type, operate machines, or drive buses. False bosoms restore women's figures. But, as one woman discovered, inflated bosoms should not be worn below 125 feet when scuba diving. She went down "a perfect 36" and surfaced flat chested—her bra had exploded.

Restoring a person's ability to function as a "total person" is a logical extension of cancer treatment that should be integrated into all hospital cancer programs, says Lawrence D. Burke, program director for Rehabilitation and Continuing Care Programs of the National Cancer Institute. "The cancer mystique, the dread, fear, and hopelessness it arouses, is responsible for many of the difficulties experienced in rehabilitating cancer patients. Yet today because of the increased survival time for cancer patients, oncologists, surgeons, and other members of the cancer treatment team minimize disability as well as treat the disease."

What a person with cancer fears most is being rejected and treated as a perpetual patient outside the hospital, in the home and on the job. Wives stop being wives and become nurses. Husbands tip-toe around the wife who has cancer. Everyone in the family has a new role to play, but unfortunately there are few stage directions for playing them.

"The husband of a woman who has cancer should not treat her as if she has changed in any way," says

Mr. Burke. "That's what she's worried about, how he thinks of her, whether she's still lovable. For a man, the diagnosis and subsequent treatment of cancer can constitute a devastating blow to his sense of masculinity. It's often a psychologically castrating experience. During the treatment period, physicians take charge of his life, the hospital fosters complete dependency and, to be a 'good patient,' personal identity and autonomy must be compromised, if not abandoned. The psychological shock requires as much rehabilitation therapy as the physical trauma."

Marriages usually undergo profound changes when one partner has cancer. In some marriages, the relationship deepens, there is a renewal of love, and a great desire for sharing. But if a relationship is shaky, the stresses of cancer can shatter it or make it almost intolerable. Even between happily married couples, there may be uncertainty about how to approach the spouse as a sexual partner. Mr. Burke's advise is for couples to "hug and kiss and fuss and fight" as they always did.

And there should be no scar secrets. Difficult as it may be for both wife and husband, they should look at the scar as soon as bandages are removed, get it over with immediately. As Mr. Burke says, the scar constitutes a part of their new physical reality, something they must see and accept.

Some hospitals have excellent cancer rehabilitation programs, many of them supported by funds from the National Cancer Institute, but this integral part of cancer treatment should be available to all cancer patients. "Rehabilitation techniques and services have been developed," says Mr. Burke, "but they are not widely applied. The need for rehabilitation therapists and for more cancer rehabilitation programs continues to increase."

There are some 350,000 people each year who, despite heroic efforts to save them, die of cancer. Some of them die without experiencing pain, but others do not. A tide of concern for those in the final stages of painful cancer has slowly arisen in America as more families were involved in the suffering and it became evident that cure-oriented hospitals were not proper settings for patients dying of cancer. The hospice concept began to take root in America.

The origins of the hospice go back to the Middle Ages when monks took in weary travelers, many of them on religious pilgrimages, deloused them, bathed and fed them, and gave them clean garments. Many pilgrims died in the hospices, not a lonely tragic experience, for in those days to die while on a religious pilgrimage meant the attainment of great spiritual rewards in the afterlife.

The modern hospice, successfully adapted in England from the medieval concept, is neither a hospital nor a nursing home. In an interview with Dr. Cicely Saunders, founder and medical director of London's famous St. Christopher's Hospice, she told me, "We visualize it as a place of hospitality where a family feeling pervades in the concern of those in charge, those who tend the patients, and those who maintain every aspect of the hospice."

The heart of the hospice program is the patient's home. In a sense the hospice is a community, encompassing patients and the staff in the building itself and patients and their families in their homes. Patients in the home care program are treated by their own family doctors and visiting nurses, but those professionals are responsible for a whole spectrum of patients—acutely ill, post-operative cases, accident victims, as well as the terminally ill. It is the patients in this last category and their families who need special skills, something extra, "compassionate friendship," extra attention at any hour when a crisis arises. The specially trained hospice staff becomes an extended family, assuaging anguish and despair, helping the patient and relatives weather emotional crises, and, after a death, sustaining the bereaved.

"We bring our patients into the hospice if there is distress which can no longer be alleviated at home when the end is near" said Dr. Saunders. "But some patients return home after the distress has been coped with. A certain number of our patients die in their own homes each year and a few are going strong contrary to the prognostications of all the doctors. Occasionally, we bring patients into the hospice to give the family some respite from the daily care of a gravely ill family member. This gives family and patients alike a chance to catch their breath, a renewal of energy and will."

In the friendly, compassionate atmosphere of the hospice, patients receive the finest medical care, backed by a staff of physicians and carefully selected and specially trained nurses, social workers, a psychiatrist, and volunteers who perform personal services for the patients. "Although the majority of patients admitted each year are dying," Dr. Saunders said, "we have long-term patients and our elderly residents, some of whom have been with us since the hospice opened in the summer of 1967. We are a mixed community with about the same number of people at home as in the hospice at any one time. And a bright, cheerful note is added by the little children of some of the staff members. When we designed the hospice, we provided for a day care center."

An ambience of hope pervades the hospice, hope of improvement that is often justified, and heartsease in the abiding covenant of care and concern. Walls of windows overlook well-tended gardens, plants line window sills, flowers are everywhere, and paintings, bold in design and color. Patients, though medicated for pain relief, are alert and ready to chat with each other or with visitors who come to the hospice from all over the world. Each patient brings some tangible link with home—a clock, photograph or picture, and occasionally a favorite chair or table. Families may visit at any time, day or night, and even bring pets. The day I was there, a family came into a ward, trailed by a huge, black Labrador dog, very well-behaved, as if it knew this was a special place. And at the bedside of his dying, young father, a little boy sat engrossed in a comic book while his father contentedly watched him.

Implicit in the modern hospice concept is that no patient suffers from pain. Instead of using the term "terminal pain," Dr. Saunders prefers the term "total pain," which, she says, includes physical and emotional pain, "social" aspects such as worries about finances or the future of young children, and those wounds of the spirit, the sense of meaninglessness and total isolation that assails so many of the dying. At St. Christopher's the patient's total pain is treated. There are no groans, no whimpers, no pain-contorted faces, no "clock watchers." Nor are there any life-extending machines, no thrumming computers or hissing respirators. "The spirit of the hospice," says Dr. Saunders, "is in its welcome for those whose lives are ending, a friendly setting where people who are dying are cared for by people who care."

Drawn to it as the model for the modern hospice, every year physicians, nurses, medical students, social workers, and health administrators make the pilgrimage to St. Christopher's. But Dr. Saunders does not consider it a model to be "slavishly" copied. Rather, she feels it should be a seedbed of ideas and concepts to be adapted.

In the United States, the hospice movement is gaining public and private support, the transplanted ideas and concepts putting down deep roots. In 1978, some 20 hospices had been opened with more in the "talking stages," and the National Hospice Organization[6] established. A direct result of White House concern for the plight of the terminally ill cancer patient was the federal Interagency Committee on New Therapies for Pain and Discomfort set up in December 1977 under the aegis of the National Institutes of Health.

President Carter's Special Assistant for Health Issues, Dr. Peter Bourne, at the second meeting of the Interagency Committee for New Therapies for Pain and Discomfort in February 1978, summarized special White House interests in these areas: facilitating research on the medicinal uses of heroin, marijuana, and other drugs; putting more emphasis on the humanitarian rather than on the technological aspects of medical care; and improving the care of the terminally ill. In regard to the last of those White House interests, Dr. Bourne expressed the hope that the federal government would play a leadership role in the hospice movement.

The National Cancer Institute has already moved in that direction, first with "seed money" of about $900,000, which helped launch Hospice, Inc., in New Haven, Connecticut, one of the first hospices in the United States. In 1978, the National Cancer Institute funded contracts for three demonstration hospice projects in New Jersey, Arizona, and California, their total funding about $4,500,000. What the Institute looks for in applications for grant funds, according to Janet L. Lunceford, R.N., who heads the Institute's hospice demonstration pro-

grams, are innovative approaches to the care of terminally ill cancer patients. "Our financial support is not
intended for hospice demonstration programs that duplicate current ones," Mrs. Lunceford says. "We are
looking for alternatives to present programs."

Dr. Kenneth Nelson, formerly associated with the
National Cancer Institute's program for continuing care
and a close observer of the hospice movement in the
United States and England, says that the English style
hospice is not feasible in the United States. "We'll develop our own style," he says. "For one thing, unlike
England, we have a scattered, heterogeneous population. Most English hospices, because in England the
Church and State are closely aligned, have a religious
overtone. That is far from the case here. And in this
country, there would be serious problems for the hospice home care program in some of our cities, especially
in high crime areas where it would be unsafe for nurses
and social workers to visit patients and their families at
all hours of the day and night. The problem in this
country in regard to hospices is not medical, but social.
Dr. Cicely Saunders at St. Christopher's and Dr. Eric
Wilkes at St. Luke's Hospice in Sheffield, England, are
tough, manager-types with charisma, and very much
admired. They would be successful in any enterprise,
superb managers and leaders. As yet in this country
we do not have that kind of leadership in the hospice
movement."

And without a National Health Service like Great
Britain's, the hospice movement in the United States
encounters a major obstacle in undefined payment
policies for medical and other services in the hospice
facility and in patients' homes. Bradley Yost, director of
Health Care Benefits for the Blue Cross Association,
looking at hospices from a "third-party" payer view-

point, cautions about developing the hospice concept without taking into account health insurance and pre-payment organizations. "Many operational hospice programs," he says, "are now receiving routine third-party reimbursement through Blue Cross and public programs for some portion of hospice care services. This is to the extent that the programs are certified or are participating providers, such as hospitals, skilled nursing facilities, home health agencies, to Medicare, Medicaid, or Blue Cross Plan programs, and that existing benefit eligibility and coverage limitations allow payment for the services rendered. Some services, however, that are essential to the hospice concept, such as family counseling, bereavement visits, and homemaker services are not typically a part of benefit coverage programs. Before there can be coverage for the full range of hospice services, there will have to be some benefit changes. Initial indications are that hospices represent a form of care with significant quality improving potential and may be cost-effective."

Commercial insurance companies, profit motivated and therefore less venturesome than Medicare and Blue Cross, will no doubt eventually extend their benefits to covering hospice services. But, according to a spokesman, such coverage will not be provided until there is more evidence of public demand for such coverage and laws and regulations are developed specifically for hospice care.

At intervals, committees meet in cities and medical centers throughout the country to talk about what might be done to alleviate the suffering of the terminally ill. Science administrators discuss ways in which illicit drugs could be licitly obtained for research on pain and distress. Insurance experts consider such matters as the cost-effectiveness of hospices and changes to be made in regulations. Among hospice advocates, well-intentioned factions emerge as they so often do among the purely motivated, and attempts are made to reconcile differences at meetings and in private discourse.

An element missing in all this diverse activity is a sense of urgency. There seems to be no awareness that while people discuss what should be done and how it might be done, loneliness, pain, and despair dominate the real world of the dying patients. A poet, David Harsent, expresses that reality in the opening line of his haunting poem, "Level 7":

The lamps of the terminal cases burn till dawn.

How long before dying cancer patients find a strong advocate who can unify the fractionated efforts on their behalf? How much longer must the lamps burn till dawn?

4 | "Painmanship"

In Victorian times, the headache was a popular form of contraception. Middle-class and rich women withdrew to their rooms. Afternoon shades were drawn. Soundproofed children tiptoed past the closed door. It was a privilege to be allowed into the room for a few moments and touch Mother's forehead with a scented handkerchief. Husbands, especially if they had mistresses and a safe quota of heirs, were solicitous, rarely insisting on conjugal rights with indisposed wives.

Georg Groddeck, credited with being the "Father" of psychosomatic medicine, considered the headache the means the unconscious uses most widely to halt thought and drive. A friend of Freud's, Groddeck took part in the tumultuous beginnings of psychiatry when theories about the unconscious dropped like bombs on the medical establishment. A physician himself, Groddeck was fascinated by the nature of illness and the possibility that there could be an unconscious will to be ill. When working up a patient's case history and considering the diagnosis, he pondered the question: What purpose could this symptom serve? In 1917, he wrote: "I consider it a basic and dangerous misconception to suppose that only the hysteric has the gift of making himself ill for whatever purpose. Every man has this

ability and each uses it in an extension beyond compre-
hension. The hysteric, and in a lesser degree the neurotic, force the observer to conclude that in being ill a
distinct purpose is served."[1]

Professional catcalls greeted Groddeck's theory.
Modestly and urbanely, he responded that he had not
expected agreement from his psychoanalytical colleagues, but he hoped his theories would at least be
tested. Fifty years later they were not merely being
tested, but applied. Behavioral scientists treating pain
patients look for the purpose the pain might serve.

In the 1960s, while visiting a pain clinic on the West
Coast, I talked with a woman patient who was undergoing a series of diagnostic tests to find the cause of the
persistent pain in her lower back. This woman, big,
spare, rawboned, and thin-lipped, was the archetypal
pioneer woman whose spine in those days somehow
survived the relentless battering of hard wood seats on
wagon trains. Though perhaps a direct descendant of
such hardy women, the woman I was talking with was
afflicted by back pain for which there seemed no physical cause. Yet she talked not about this persistent pain,
but about her two sons, soldiers fighting in Vietnam.
They were real men, she said proudly, not like those
conscientious objectors who were too cowardly to
fight. Though she said nothing derogatory about her
husband, it was quite evident from her facial expression
and her tone of voice that his two wonderful sons far
outclassed him.

She had worked hard all her life, she told me, managing a big house, raising the two boys, tending the large
vegetable garden. Now that both sons were gone, she
and her husband had moved into a smaller house and
she had managed the whole operation, packing and
unpacking and settling things as they should be. But not

long after they had moved into the house, she began to get backaches that prevented her doing housework or gardening, though it was a much smaller garden than before. She couldn't even drive the car, her back hurt so much. Her husband had to take time off from work to drive her fifty miles to the pain clinic.

Oddly, this woman in her fifties, partially disabled by back pain, was wearing three-inch-high spike heels. Later, when I attended the pain treatment team's discussion of her case, the psychologist and the social worker pinpointed without much difficulty the purpose of this woman's undiagnosed pain—with her sons gone, she had no incentive for maintaining house and garden and husband. She had done everything for years, now it was his turn.

Dr. Thomas Szasz, psychiatrist, coined the word *painmanship* to indicate the use of pain for some advantage. In what he calls the "communicative meaning" of pain, Dr. Szasz says in *Pain and Pleasure* that it is a way of asking for help, consciously when someone cries out, or more subtly in a silent appeal to a particular person. The person suffering may not actually need the help of that person or even expect it, yet makes the appeal because of a feeling that something is owed to him, some payment of justly earned dues.

In his psychiatric practice, Dr. Szasz found that patients with pain problems rarely seek his help on their own initiative, but because they have been referred by physicians. Unable to relate their physical pain to emotional and psychological difficulties, these reluctant patients attribute it to some physical cause their doctor cannot discover. Characteristic of these patients is that many of them have coped very well with minor, often sporadic pain, but overwhelmed by some emotional crisis, seek help for the pain.

Several things about these patients puzzle Dr. Szasz. Why is it that though they complain of pain, they show no sign of tension, no pallor, or other clue in facial expression? Why do these patients feel pain in the absence of demonstrable disease or injury? Why does the pain persist? What is the meaning of the mutually frustrated and hostile patient-doctor interaction usually present in this type of situation?

A patient may be saying: "I need help. The pressures on me are too much for me to bear and I have no one else to turn to." Or, "I can no longer endure being disregarded." What the patient may be demanding silently is: "Pay attention to me!" You see it in offices, in any work place, the complainer who answers even the morning ritual question, "How're you?" with a full medical report—the sleepless night, postnasal drip in the morning, stiff knees, sore back. This self-defeating device for sympathy and attention, after a while, usually results not in transfixed attention, but in people never asking: "How're you?"

Not everyone shies away from these people. Some sufferers get an added, vicarious thrill out of the pain and suffering of others. Eyes aglitter, they gloat on details, swap information about various pain-relieving drugs, exchange analgesics, and send each other clippings of news stories on discoveries of new painkillers. For every minor symptom, they have a fatal diagnosis. Almost a requirement for being accepted in certain social clusters of older people is that you have a disorder you are willing to talk about. In these groups there are hierarchies of medical problems, surgery at the pinnacle, bunions at the bottom. Any elderly person who has no ailments, who has other things to talk about, may be subtly ostracized by his or her own age group. It's as if pain, suffering, and distress were initiation fees.

Men and women have found that, in order to belong, they must adhere to the aching, suffering stereotype.

Using pain as an attention getter can backfire with the medical profession, as Dr. I. Pilowsky points out in his article, "The Psychiatrist and the Pain Clinic."[2] Dr. Pilowsky, a professor of psychiatry at the University of Adelaide in Australia, says that the patient whose pain is associated with guilt feelings of loss, anger, or dependence makes demands on and achieves a close relationship with a host of professionals. But if a patient with these guilt feelings repeatedly complains of pain to clinicians who do not understand the significance and function of the pain, he inevitably provokes in the physicians anxiety, anger, and guilt. "These responses may in turn lead to covert and overt attacks on the patient," says Dr. Pilowsky. "Covert attacks may include painful investigations and operations, and overt ones may involve quite frank castigation of the patient and the imputation of malingering, lying, or mental illness. A reaction of this sort on the clinician's part must inevitably result in a hostile response from the patient, coupled with fear of total rejection."

A familiar figure in the pain clinic is the hypochondriac who, as Thornton Wilder said, "listens to his body as if it were a Stradivarius." The faintest twinge, the slightest hint that something is out of tune sends him searching for medical aid and reassurance. Body-listeners use pain as an enduring solution for other problems. It conceals loneliness, the void left when an aged parent who had been the focus of love and care dies and leaves a daughter or son who cannot fill the void except with suffering. Pain can be a mask for rebellion against a jaded marriage. It's quite acceptable for a woman to admit to other women that her husband is a rascal and a womanizer, but rarely does she publicly admit that he is a bore. Such an accusation would be "putting on airs," making herself out to be better than wives who hadn't noticed how boring their own husbands were. But she gets inverted sympathy from those same women who can understand physical but not intellectual suffering. Who knows how many car and motorcycle smashups occur as young people expiate their sense of guilt over disappointing their parents who worked hard and sacrificed much to pay for their education? People face problems today that a century ago death spared them. Men who died in the early fifties had no time to worry about the loss of youthful vigor and sexual prowess. Nor were there the dilemmas about what to do with aging parents—they remained in the household. Nor did they worry about getting cancer. In our time the stress of unresolved emotional problems, so many so difficult to solve, wraps us in a blanket of pain, insulates us from nagging guilt and anxiety that, compared to them, is easier to bear.

Animals of all sorts, including man, have been induced to accomplish almost impossible tasks under the lash, the slave and the lash being inseparable from ancient times to the mid-1900s. But another type of pain harder to rebel against is that portrayed in Edith Wharton's story, *Ethan Frome*. A bitter, suffering woman, crippled in a botched, double-suicide attempt instigated by her lover, reduces him to a servant, using his guilt as her weapon. Wives use chronic pain to revenge themselves on philandering husbands. Children quite early learn how to manipulate indifferent parents through pain. And in the work place, scores are settled. The typist who despises her illiterate boss, the assistant manager who had all the good ideas but never got the credit, the worker who cleans the toilets, all find ways of getting out of their jobs and onto the disability rolls.

In small towns, there are the disability pensioners, envied by some, despised by others, who report on intermittent pain just often enough to justify their status. And there is the living saint, the woman who patiently endures suffering, an inspiration, as her minister so often tells her, to the entire community. A devoted husband waits on her hand and foot, "a marvelous man." Surprisingly, quite a few bedridden wives are miraculously cured by the death of those devoted husbands, quit their beds of pain, and take over the chairmanship of the church supper committee.

Pain ranks almost with money in the power it invests people with to tyrannize over others. The father whose rotten disposition must be forever excused because his back hurts. You've seen those mother-daughter pairs at church and in the supermarket, the elderly mother walking painfully, leaning heavily on the daughter's arm and the daughter in her unhappy, single middle age, the nurse her mother gave birth to and reared. And the man who transforms a whiplash injury into a way of life, keeping his family in an uproar with endless court battles over disability compensation payments that are never enough.

Most treasured among rewards of the pain game is confounding doctors. The greater the doctor's reputation, the greater the triumph. This type of pain patient-surgeon transaction falls into the category Dr. Eric Berne[3] identifies with the acronym NIGYYSOB ("Now I've Got You, You Son of a Bitch"). In this type of pain game, players suffering from chronic, undiagnosed pain make the rounds of prominent surgeons until they find one who can be cajoled into believing that only he with his marvelous skill can perform the operation that will cure the pain. No matter that five other topflight surgeons have failed to cure this patient's pain. (Even surgeons have days when their wits are not so sharp as their scalpels.) The great surgeon agrees to operate.

The patient experiences the satisfactions of surgical foreplay—boasting to friends that the distinguished surgeon has accepted him or her as a patient, recounting details of the initial interview, the presurgical tests, some more painful than the chronic pain itself. And the ineffable excitements of surgery—attention from doctors and nurses, flowers and cards, phone calls, visitors. The patient squeezes every advantage out of the experience and three months later tells the great surgeon he has failed. The pain has not been cured. The surgeon is defeated, another victim to the NIGYYSOB game.

A variation of the pain game is the my-pain-is-worse-than-yours, a game usually played by husband and wife. He gets a pain in the chest; she gets a worse one in the stomach. He gets chills and fever; she gets pneumonia. He wrenches his back moving the sofa; she sprains her ankle playing tennis. Between husband and wife it's a harmless enough game, but when a parent plays it with children, competing with them for attention and sympathy, the game acquires neurotic overtones.

Pain is part of love games. Partners flay each other, bite, pinch, scratch, and inflict pain and injuries that in a barroom brawl would lead to the arrest of the participants. In Ann Landers's newspaper column, a window on American mores, men and women readers have defended flagellation as a stimulating version of sexual foreplay, in some instances essential for arousal. (Miss Landers does not approve of it.)

No one forgets those early years of life when, as an attractive, lovable baby, one was the object of affectionate smiles, pats, kisses, and hugs. There are those who say we spend the rest of our lives trying to recapture that love, never forgetting those sensations. Not even the very elderly forget the sensations of love. In his poem, "Persuasions to Love," Thomas Carew says:

> When beauty, youth and all sweets leave her,
> Love may return, but lover never;
> And old folks say there are no pains
> Like itch of love in aged veins.

Psychologists and physicians specializing in pain management have discovered that some pain-prone patients are remarkably similar to the classic accident-prone type. Both are repeaters. The accident-prone type manages to fall down stairs, trip over rugs, burn his hands on hot handles, and injure himself in a series of accidents that most other people seem able to avoid. The pain-prone type has been repeatedly disabled by pain, though there may be no visible lesions or evidence of injury to account for the pain. Most of these people are surgery addicts, collecting scars, but not relief. Their personalities are described as resentful and hostile. They tend to blame their suffering on malevolent fate or on someone close to them.

Dr. Richard Sternbach in some of his studies found that these people are very likely to come from homes in which aggression and pain figured prominently. Generally, their parents were cold and indifferent, even cruel, and showed concern only when the children were sick or injured. Because the only sign that the parents "cared" was through abuse, pain became associated with the recognition of the child's existence, if only as an object of anger. Later on, in adult life, some of these emotionally warped people use their own pain as an instrument of self-abuse.

And the parents who engendered this distorted behavior in their children later on can become pathetically sentimental about them. Erasing cleanly recollections of the cruel treatment they inflicted on their wretched children, marring them for life, these parents make a great show of family ties. These are the parents who use the telephone line as a sort of umbilical cord wrapped around their distant children. Children who were physically punished, not as part of the normal teaching pattern but as objects of uncontrollable wrath and viciousness, later get back at their parents with cold indifference, settling the score decades later. Sometimes, though, instead of settling the score with their parents, they take their buried rage and grief out on their own children. And the terrible cycle continues.

The most practical reward of pain is financial. Most people injured on the job, in a friend's house, or in traffic accidents will settle for reasonable amounts if there is nothing extraordinary about the circumstances, like a drunk driver smashing into a car. But often egged on by lawyers who collect a large percentage of the financial award, accident victims have been suing for more and more money, some for outrageous sums. Abuse of the compensation system is so widespread that doctors are suspicious of patients on disability. And in some communities, the doctors themselves are part of the conspiracy. Perhaps the worst penalty of overblown suits for compensation is that the promise of financial rewards makes liars and deceivers out of otherwise decent people.

A devastating reward of persistent pain is drug addiction. Without any way of measuring pain, physicians cannot judge whether chronic pain has persisted for months or years without any apparent reason. They must believe the patient who says, "I can't stand it, doctor. You'll have to give me something." It is remarkable how little is known about medically induced drug addiction. It seems not to arouse the interest of the massive federal antiaddiction effort which is primarily aimed at socially disadvantaged drug addicts.

The American attitude was set as far back as 1901 in a Senate resolution which prohibited the sale by American traders of opium and alcohol to "aboriginal tribes and uncivilized races," a resolution later extended to include "uncivilized elements in America itself and its territories, such as Indians, Alaskans, the inhabitants of Hawaii, railroad workers, and immigrants at port of entry." The target group now is young people, especially young blacks.

But affluent adults who get their addictive drugs by prescription are singularly free from harassment and jail sentences. You have never seen a front-page story (with pictures) about drug law-enforcement agents raiding a local hospital to round up physicians and nurses who are drug addicts—yet there are many who are. No pain clinic will be raided and newly arrived patients still on their addictive drug schedules, not yet weaned, picked up and carted away in police patrol wagons. Yet many pain specialists at clinics estimate that 50 percent of patients arrive addicted to narcotic and other types of analgesics. The first phase of pain clinic treatment is usually to reduce drug dependence, sometimes "cold turkey" or sometimes by a gradual process as emphasis is shifted to pain management techniques and behavior changes. A curious but not uncommon phenomenon is that, once off the drugs, many patients discover that they no longer have the pain for which the drugs were originally prescribed. The drug game often supersedes the pain game.

There are no real winners in the pathetic, destructive game of painmanship. But as the rewards of pain become better understood and the alternatives to game playing more widely used by pain specialists, the game will attract fewer players. The corollary to Dr. Groddeck's theory that people can make themselves ill is: People using that same indefinable power can make themselves well.

5 | from Witch Doctors to Endorphins

When we talk about pain we usually mean the feeling we have when we hurt physically. The English word *pain* comes from the Latin *poena,* meaning penalty or punishment. Small wonder, with such a root, that the experience of pain is enshrouded in an aura of guilt and superstition. In its long journey from classical to modern times, the word has picked up other meanings: lost love, "hurt feelings" evoked by unkind words or snubs, toil, and mental anguish.

As many-faceted as a rose-cut diamond, pain has as many interpretations as there are subjective and objective points of view. To someone who feels it, pain hurts. Physicians view it as a warning or, if it serves no such purpose, as a disease in itself. Parents use pain to discipline. Theologians preach its spiritual values. To sociologists, pain and the threat of it are powerful tools for survival. Behavioral scientists consider it an experience that can be modified and one that is influenced by personality, rewards, life goals, and cultural tradition. Of special interest to psychiatrists is pain of psychogenic origins. Scientists are intrigued by its mechanisms and new chemical and surgical ways for controlling it.

Paranoid from the very beginning, man attributed his inexplicable catastrophes to malevolent spirits, vengeful, bad-tempered, vain, but amenable to negotiations. Spirits could be bribed by sacrifices, incantations, and elaborate rituals in their honor. But when he found he wasn't making much headway placating evil spirits— lightning still struck, the roof of his cave fell in, and his body was repeatedly assailed by torments—he hit upon the idea of an intercessor, the "witch doctor" who had special powers of communication with the spirits. Medicine men gradually acquired power over body and spirit, their status raised in ancient times to that of priest.

"The campaign against pain got under way only when body and soul were divorced by Descartes," says Ivan Illich in *Medical Nemesis*. "He constructed an image of the body in terms of geometry, mechanics or watchmaking, a machine that could be repaired by an engineer. . . . For Descartes pain became a signal with which the body reacts in self-defense to protect its mechanical integrity. These reactions to danger are transmitted to the soul, which recognizes them as painful. Pain was reduced to a useful learning device: it now taught the soul how to avoid further damage to the body." Descartes advanced his theory of the separation of body and soul in the early seventeenth century, opening the way for modern medical science.

Before science came to his aid, man had assuaged his sufferings with prayers, talismans, drugs, herbs and roots, and other growing things, among them the poppy, mandragora, hemp, and henbane. As early as 2250 b.c., a Babylonian clay tablet records a remedy for toothache. Ancient man used opium, surgery, heat, cold, and massage to relieve pain, even electrotherapy for neuralgia and headache by ingeniously applying the supercharged torpedo fish to the aching part. About 200 a.d., the physician Galen advocated opium and mandragora as well as electrotherapy for control of pain. During the Dark Ages when medicine in Europe suffered an eclipse, medicine's center of gravity shifted to Arabia where the physician Avicenna made a special contribution to the understanding of pain by describing some fifteen different types of it and ways of alleviating them, suggestions that became medical guidelines for six centuries.

In medieval times the question "Why me?" was not so common as it is today. People then knew quite well why they had been singled for pain and suffering. The Church made it eminently clear: They were miserable sinners, marked by sin even before they were born. At that time when very little could be done to find and correct the cause of pain and its warning value was nugatory, religious faith supplied some degree of assuagement, the knowledge that the suffering was not in vain, that it would be recognized in the final tally. Religious relics, aided by intense faith and hope, worked miraculous cures. If, however, cures were not forthcoming, then the sufferer should look to his conscience. In any case, no one asked for his money back or sued the Church. Prayers, pilgrimages, crusades, gold, and property given in God's name to churches, all played their role in the ceaseless search for nepenthe.

In the nineteenth century, opium was the aspirin of the people. Cheap and easy to come by, available at any apothecary, and, at that time, free of social stigma, opium was the analgesic of choice for workmen and the gentry. Sylvester Gilbert, a Connecticut lawyer, writing to his granddaughter in 1839, thanked her for sending "the medications, including opium, which were welcome for various ailments and as a tranquilizer." Laudanum, a liquid form of opium, was a popular remedy for toothache, a remedy that Thomas De Quincey, after becoming addicted to it, alternately extolled and reproached.

Until the discovery of anesthesia in the nineteenth century, pain as a warning served a limited purpose. Though surgery might be indicated, only the hardy and heroic survived the indescribable pain and shock as surgeons, stalwart as their patients, cut into fully conscious, thrashing patients who were restrained by thick leather straps and burly attendants. Unless a patient had the luck to faint, he experienced agonizing pain, exacerbated by the rasping sound of a saw severing a bone. In those circumstances, operations were marvels of skill, speed, and brute strength, though few patients survived to appreciate their contribution to those surgical triumphs.

A portrait of the first surgical team to use anesthesia on a patient hangs in the Harvard University Medical School. Grouped around the patient are doctors dressed as if on their way to present diplomatic credentials to a foreign power. If patients survived the surgery, their next obstacle to recovery was the germs their saviors brought with them into the operating room.

Though anesthesia eased matters for patients and surgeons during amputations, abdominal surgery needed another scientific advance to make it feasible. When the taut abdominal muscles holding internal organs in place are cut, the organs spill out. The solution came not from a laboratory initially, but from South American jungles. Explorers returning from the jungles reported on a poison named curare that primitive natives used on the tips of their arrows. When a poison-tipped arrow penetrated skin, the curare caused total relaxation of the body's systemic functions and subsequent death. Medical scientists experimented with the

strange substance and developed safe doses that relaxed muscles enough for surgery, but allowed the functions of the body to continue. From then on physical
strength in surgery was replaced by clever, deft hands.

During the nineteenth century, while clinical progress
was being made on the conquest of pain, a parallel development was taking place in laboratories where scientists spent much time thinking. In 1811, the Scottish
physiologist Sir Charles Bell theorized that the skin had
specific receptors for the sensations of cold, heat, touch,
and pain. It was the first of many theories that would be
argued among scientists for the next 166 years, argu-
ments still going on. But it opened the way for thinking
about pain in a rational way, putting it in a category
as an entity. Theories that a special apparatus for pain
existed in the body were strongly opposed. New theories were proposed.

What was generally agreed upon was that pain was a
reaction against tissue damage, a protective reaction,
something to make an animal avoid damaging contact,
but one that would also suppress these reactions under
certain circumstances. The man or other animal injured
in a life-threatening situation must be able to disregard
the pain and flee. In other words, the automatic reactions must be kept subservient to the primary goal of
survival. An animal caught in a trap will gnaw off its
paw to escape. A man who has broken a leg jumping
from a burning building will hobble or crawl away from
the fire.

As theories of pain mechanisms were developed,
neurosurgeons adapted techniques to take advantage
of them. One of the first was the cordotomy, cutting the
spinal cord along which pain messages travel. The pain
below the incision disappeared. But after a while, pain
returned, and, strangely enough, a pain of a different

quality. Dorsal column stimulators were implanted for back pain. Again the results were limited to a short time, and unforeseen complications, such as hemorrhage in the spinal cord, revealed the risks of the operation.

Every surgical technique to interfere with pain pathways in the spinal cord is hazardous, and in some instances pain resulting from the surgery can be more devastating than the original pain. As Dr. John A. Jane, head of neurosurgery at the University of Virginia School of Medicine, has said, "Our efforts should be devoted, even accentuated to trying to solve the problem of pain in terms of looking at basic mechanisms and trying to understand them. As a clinician, I'm pessimistic right now. As a scientist, I'm very optimistic that this fascinating problem can be looked at effectively in the laboratory."[1]

In 1965, two scientists announced a new theory of the mechanisms of pain that, like none before it, set off a wave of basic research and clinical application. Dr. Ronald Melzack, psychophysiologist, teamed up with Dr. Patrick Wall, a neurophysiologist, to develop the spinal-gate theory. This pairing of psychology, physiology, and neuroanatomy in pain mechanism research gave scientists a new, broader insight into the nature of pain. Briefly, the Melzack-Wall theory postulates that, in nerves composed of different size fibers, the larger fibers transmit impulses related to touch, while the smaller ones, which conduct impulses more slowly, transmit pain impulses. Both sets of nerves converge in the spinal cord. It is at this convergence point that, according to the theory, the gate mechanism exists.

As Dr. Melzack explains the theory: "When signals for moderate sensations like itching or a slight burn are transmitted along the small fibers, the gate remains partially open. If a sensation is intensified, more small fibers become active and carry pain messages through the gate to the brain. However, activity in the large fibers, produced by rubbing or scratching, tends to close the gate and block itching and pain. Pain messages are also modulated by emotional factors—anxiety, pleasure, hope. These messages move down from the brain to the gate and act on the pain signals. Negative emotions such as anxiety, fear, or sadness open the gate to pain impulses; joy, exhilaration, and expectation close it, at least for a time."

The new theory touched off debates that twelve years later were still raging. As Dr. Melzack says in "The Gate Theory Revisited,"[2] "New biological-medical theories, like theories in the physical sciences, are accepted reluctantly; an old theory is dogmatically maintained in the face of contrary evidence until a new theory that can account for both the older and newer facts supersedes it. In this process of evolution, there is usually a characteristic swing of the pendulum between two major theoretical concepts until one eventually dominates . . . a theory may be *conceptually* correct although the particular explanatory *mechanism* that is postulated may well be wrong in one or more details.

"Overriding all of these features of the scientific process is the bitter controversy generated between opposing schools of thought. The problems of cutaneous mechanisms in general, and pain in particular, have given rise to vituperation that is unparalleled in the biological sciences. . . . Part of the reason for the bitterness engendered by the battle may be the obvious clinical implications that derive from any theoretical advance. The practice of medicine, because it deals with human lives, is generally conservative; so old ideas that have worked (even imperfectly) are cherished and newer ideas are viewed with suspicion and often antipathy."

Dr. Melzack's conclusions about the gate-control theory in 1977, twelve years after it was published, are that it "is alive and well despite considerable controversy and conflicting evidence" and the need for some physiological details. Research based on the theory shows that the descending control over the gate is extremely powerful and that intense stimulation is capable of inhibiting pain signals "and may represent an important clinical approach to the modulation of pain."

The gate-control theory of pain, besides stimulating a vast amount of research, says Dr. Melzack, "has played a major role in the recognition of pain as a medical syndrome in its own right, rather than merely a symptom of other pathological processes. The development of pain clinics for the treatment of pain has occurred hand-in-hand with the burgeoning research, and both have revealed new facets of the puzzle of pain. . . . Even the effects of acupuncture on some kinds of chronic pain are put into focus within the framework of the gate theory. They are no longer seen as mysterious, but simply as an example of the modulation of pain by sensory input."

The Melzack-Wall theory provides an explanation of the limitless influences on our interpretation of pain. Age is one factor—children's tolerance is generally far below that of adults. Other factors are race, physical condition (athletes manage pain much better than the rest of us), social training, religious bias, attention, the state of a disease, suggestion, time of day or night, weather, the likely duration of pain (the quick jab of the inoculation needle contrasted with the endless duration of intractable pain), and the purpose the pain serves (the mother giving birth to the child, the long-distance runner out front and heading for the tape).

An area of pain control being rigorously pursued by scientists as a result of the Melzack-Wall gate theory is finding new ways of noninjurious counterstimulation. It has been known for some time that one pain can inhibit another, called the pain paradox and a concept underlying acupuncture. Not yet explained is why the primary pain is often permanently relieved by the stimulation of the applied pain. A theory that might explain chronic pain is that a normal function of the gray matter in the brainstem in inhibiting excessive central nervous system activity fails to work, thereby allowing continuous pain messages to be transmitted. Another intensely painful stimulus might trigger the defective control system, get it working again, and control the pain.

On the heels of the Melzack-Wall theory came the electrifying discovery of opiate receptors in the brain. Dr. Candace Pert and Dr. Solomon Snyder of Johns Hopkins University School of Medicine, in the course of their studies on drug addiction, found that morphine, heroin, and other opium derivatives attach to certain brain cell sites, called receptors, into which the narcotic drugs fit like keys into their proper locks. The presence of these opiate receptors indicated that, in the evolution of man and other animals, these receptors served some important function and that they had existed for millions of years before the discovery of opium.

Why, scientists asked, does the brain have a receptor for a plant that few animals come in contact with? Was it possible that the body produced a natural substance that had the pain-relieving properties of opiates? These questions touched off an international race among scientists to find such a substance in animals. Only a year after the discovery of the opiate receptors in 1973, the race was won by Dr. John Hughes and his associates at the University of Aberdeen in Scotland. The scientists reported that they had extracted from laboratory animals a chemical (which they named enkephalin) similar to morphine that bound to the opiate receptors in the same manner as opiates. When injected into the brains of laboratory rats, the newly discovered natural substance had pain-suppressing effects.

In quick succession, researchers isolated variations of enkephalin, one named endorphin, released by the pituitary gland, that is a natural pain suppressor 200 times more powerful than morphine. Aside from the incalculable possibilities for pain relief implied in this research, and the fantastical discovery that man is born with his own supply of narcotics, these exciting developments give pain research a higher status in the snob-ridden scientific hierarchy. A well-timed, generous infusion of research funds from federal agencies would attract young, adventurous scientists into the field.

Information on the mechanisms of endorphins has already led to studies of their relation to acupuncture, a pain control method disdained in some scientific circles because its mechanisms are not understood. (No one knows how aspirin works either.) Dr. Bruce Pomerantz of the University of Toronto has demonstrated that acupuncture slows the rate at which certain cells in the brain fire in response to pain. After he removed an anesthetized animal's pituitary gland, acupuncture had no pain-relieving effect, indicating that in some way acupuncture stimulates the release of the body's pain suppressor, its natural opiate. Research on the mechanism of hypnosis, another successful "spook" method of pain control, indicates that endorphins play a role in its effects. Pharmaceutical company scientists, taking up the search for a synthetic form of enkephalin, have already developed a related chemical substance that has pain-suppressing effects in animals.

Some scientists are skeptical about the body's pain-suppression system. But others are sufficiently convinced to make this line of investigation one of the fastest moving in biomedical research. Ultimately scientists hope to find ways of stimulating man's natural pain-suppression system and to develop synthetic enkephalin that will be as effective as opiate analgesics without their addictive qualities.

For decades scientists have been trying to develop synthetic painkillers that have the benefits of morphine without its drawbacks. Preeminent among these scientists is Dr. Everette May, formerly of the National Institutes of Health, who described in an interview the characteristics of an ideal painkiller: "In general, we look for a drug that takes effect quickly, has long duration of action and, of course, one that has minimal side effects, such as respiratory depression, nausea, and drug dependence, and that can be as effective taken through the mouth as by injection."

Morphine is the analgesic preferred by doctors, though according to Dr. May, it is not by any means the most effective or the most potent. "There are many drugs more potent than morphine and probably some better ones, but it, along with Demerol, is most frequently used. Doctors prefer morphine because they have used it for years. They know what it will do and what to expect from it and many are loath to change to a new and perhaps more effective drug."

In developing a new synthetic analgesic, Dr. May and his associates first look at the chemical structure of a drug like morphine and sort out what they think are the features responsible for its painkilling action. Then with simple chemical blocks, they build as simple a molecule as possible. Once the compound has been synthesized, it is tested in mice for pain relief.

In the laboratory, a technician takes two or three mice out of a jar containing a small colony of mice. The ones I saw were snowy white, appealing little creatures with tiny pink jade eyes and delicate, almost transparent pink feet. After they were given a shot of the synthetic analgesic, they were put on a hot plate. As the heat increased, the technician watched the mice's feet. When a rear foot was raised, it signaled that the mouse felt the heat. The mouse was taken off the hot plate and the time from injection of the analgesic to the lifting of the foot was recorded. In the next test, the pain stimulus is electrical impulses to the base of the mouse's tail which is held firmly by a large plastic clothespin containing electrodes. Voltages are increased until the mouse squeaks three times. No one knows why three squeaks is the mouse's signal of pain perception and scientists do not question the validity of that signal, for as one scientist says: "Who ever heard of a stoic mouse?" After the three squeaks, the time is recorded, and the mouse returned to the glass jar.

The next test is in monkeys. If the new compound passes that test, it is ready to be tested on human beings. New synthetics used to be tested on prisoners at the federal government's Addiction Research Center in Lexington, Kentucky, but, since the government now prohibits using prisoners in research studies, that phase of the testing has been halted. Scientists are looking for research model substitutes for human beings. Before a new synthetic can be produced and marketed by a pharmaceutical company, it must get approval from the Food and Drug Administration. In all, the process takes as much as seven or more years from the first experiments with the chemical building blocks to the sale of the drug.

Besides being put off by the complexities of analgesic research, many scientists are reluctant to conduct tests of analgesics on patients that require withholding pain relief from a control group of sufferers in order to measure the effects of the drug on another group in the study. Other scientists shy away from research in which animals are subjected to induced pain. It is, of course, unpardonable to keep a laboratory animal in constant severe pain in order to study it.

Quite a few agencies collect large sums from the public to protect animals from being subjected to painful experiments. Representatives of these agencies descend on the National Institutes of Health now and then and scrutinize research grant applications, looking for evidence of studies in which animals endure painful procedures. Oddly, there has never been an indignant delegation to the National Institutes of Health demanding that something be done about the suffering of human beings.

The most dynamic pain research program in the Public Health Service is conducted by the National Institute on Drug Abuse, not an agency you would expect to have a primary interest in the subject. But that institute, in connection with its aim of finding a base for understanding the nature of addiction and its management, in 1977 funded 54 pain-related research projects, most on the mechanisms of pain and on analgesia. "Support of research in these areas," says Dr. Lorenz K. Y. Ng of the institute's Division of Research, "has already opened up several new and exciting areas of investigation. It has spurred current studies on the nature of the opiate receptors and the endogenous morphine-like factors, endorphins, areas of investigation which are on the frontiers of narcotic addiction research today."

The institute took the lead in studies of the effectiveness of heroin in the treatment of terminal cancer patients. In 1977, it awarded to the Sloan-Kettering Institute in New York City a $1,200,000 grant for a 5-year research program on several analgesic drugs, including heroin. The heroin study, said Dr. Ng, "will examine the relative analgesic potency of heroin and will study the time course of action of heroin, morphine, meperidine, and methadone. The studies will also examine the levels of endorphins in human cerebro-spinal fluid and the effects of endorphins in patients with pain. Endorphin levels will be measured in several categories of patients in pain."

Dr. Ng and his associates are conducting studies of chemical, physiological, and psychological factors related to pain, measuring them before and after patients with chronic pain have received pain control treatment, including transcutaneous stimulation and electrical acupuncture. "Too little is known about chronic pain," said Dr. Ng. "While acute pain may have a useful function as a symptom of an underlying pathology or illness, chronic pain seems to have negative survival value. As a maladaptive function, it should be treated as a primary problem rather than a symptom, an important point physicians often do not understand. In my opinion, the chronic pain patient shares many similarities with the narcotic addict, including their high rate of relapse. Despite their complaints of discomfort, many chronic pain patients are in a true sense addicted to their pain. In their behavioral dependency problems, they share many similar features with those of the narcotic addict.

A better understanding of ways to treat and manage chronic pain as a primary problem could shed light on ways of treating and managing narcotic addiction."

In the 1960s when the behavioral scientists joined the search for ways of controlling pain, a truly multidisciplinary approach was launched and solutions to the pain problem never looked brighter.

6 | the Pain Pit

A 49-year-old Pennsylvania construction worker injured his foot in an automobile accident. Arthritis set in and three years after the accident, unable to endure the pain any longer, he shot off his foot.

There are no measurements of desperation until afterwards, when the evidence is self-mutilation or suicide. Even in hospitals where patients are carefully monitored some patients find ways of killing themselves when pain becomes intolerable. Not that medical professionals are inhuman, but in the hospital system, pain relief has a low priority.

The modern hospital is a work place where skilled people perform tasks within a system as tightly organized as an industrial plant. The end product of the system is a cured person. To this end, whatever contributes to cure is justifiable: diagnostic tests and treatment methods sometimes more distressing—and dangerous—than the disease or injury.

In this cure-oriented setting, suffering is a by-product, regrettable, but necessary. Patients are expected to control their expressions of pain, the groans, cries, or whimpering that upset the staff, agitate other patients, and disturb the disciplined mood of the ward. For certain procedures such as having dead tissue removed from burns or giving birth to a child, there are acceptable levels of pain expressions, but patients who exceed those levels are labeled uncooperative or difficult.

In a study of patient-staff interactions in pain management, investigators[1] found that when "expected pain trajectories" are unusual, relations between patients and staff deteriorate. "Psychiatrists are then frequently called —but to no avail, either because it is too late to break the vicious cycle of worsening relationships, or because they do not understand the complexities of the work situation. As a consequence, the nursing and sometimes the medical care of these patients tends to suffer."

The study showed that patients with chronic disease have an especially bad time of it in hospitals. Many chronic pain patients before entering the hospital were accustomed to taking pain medications in specific doses at definite times. In the hospital, the staff takes over pain management and, in some instances, without consulting either the patient or physician, changes the pain medication and the schedule for administering it. "Several patients," say the investigators, "told us that they warned nurses and physicians about specific drugs which they knew to be ineffective or to trigger allergic reactions, only to have their warnings ignored. . . ."

To a dying man or woman, a painful procedure may not seem advantageous, but to the hospital staff it is part of the patient's medical management. These differing points of view further strain patient-staff relations, creating antagonism, staff withdrawal, rejection, and sometimes the departure of the patient from the hospital. In their report of this study, the investigators say that current practices of pain management in hospitals show it to be peripheral in the staff's opinion to their attention and responsibilities. "And by responsibilities we mean not merely the staff's perceived responsibilites, but their actual legal and organizational ones. We are asserting, in other words, that *the staff is not genuinely accountable for much of its interaction with or behavior toward patients in pain.* . . . Until staff become genuinely accountable for their pain work, there will be little improvement in the care of the patients."

Appeals for pain relief to family physicians by hospitalized patients or by their relatives may be fruitless, for once his patients are in the hospital, the doctor becomes part of the system. In that highly organized setting, the doctor's informal office manner is transformed by an aura of authority. A figure of power and pressing responsibilities, he comes briskly into a patient's room, rarely sits down to ask questions that would reveal the patient's condition beyond what is written on the chart, whether, for instance, pain prevents sleeping, or moving, or eating, or whether the pain medication is sufficient to keep ahead of the pain. The patient, grateful for the doctor's visit, anxious to put on a brave show for the busy professional, generally represses the truth about hurting, rarely tells about sleepless nights, watching the illuminated hands of the bedside clock crawl toward the next dose of pain medication. (*Clock watchers* is the term used by the staff for these patients.)

Inadequate pain control in hospitals is also due to physicians' lack of information about drug options and combinations, and misjudging the duration of analgesic action. The hysteria about drug addiction rubs off on physicians, especially in the hospital setting where whatever he or she does is scrutinized by the staff. In private practice when treating chronic pain, physicians are less cautious. As directors of pain clinics know, the first step in treatment very often is weaning patients from addictive drugs.

Dr. Thomas P. Hackett, chief of psychiatric consultant

services at Massachusetts General Hospital, suspects that some doctors are influenced by their own prejudices in regard to patients in pain. In his article, "Pain and Prejudice,"[2] Dr. Hackett says that many physicians still believe that to be real, pain must have an organic cause. They regard psychogenic pain suspiciously. Disregarding the wide alterations of pain experience even in the same individual, they consider the presence or absence of organic pathology the determining factor in how a person reacts to pain under different circumstances. "By using acute pain as the model for all pain, they fail to take into account the ways people adapt to pain of long duration and their ability to control their expression of it even though discomfort may be intense. Successful adaptation, not showing the usual signs of pain, not giving expected clues undermines a doctor's belief that a patient's pain exists."

Another prejudice cited by Dr. Hackett is the use of narcotics in the treatment of pain. "By and large, narcotics are dispensed with little consideration for the patient. We have standard doses that are rarely altered to accommodate discrepancies in body weight and even less frequently are allowances made for an individual's drug tolerances. While it is true that narcotics are dangerous drugs which depress cell metabolism and addict certain people, their primary purpose is to provide effective relief from pain. This is sometimes lost sight of."

Down at the bottom of the pain pit are patients hospitalized for treatment of chronic low back pain, an ambiguous, not life-threatening condition devoid of any medical panache. Low back pain sets off no galvanizing response in hospital staff members.

Yet Dr. Bernard E. Finneson,[3] who specializes in treating low back pain, says back problems are "the worst plague of the twentieth century," afflicting an estimated

20 to 40 million Americans. Years ago, it was mostly elderly people who developed back trouble, usually after years of hard work on farms, in forests, and on the docks. Now, back problems afflict the young as well as the elderly.

It's the way we live, Dr. Finneson says. Immobilized behind desks, driving instead of walking, slumping for hours in overstuffed chairs watching television, we suddenly stress unused back muscles in a vigorous tennis game, skiing down mountains, moving the television set from one room to another, reaching out from the car seat to pull shut a heavy door, even changing a tire. Among young people, car crashes account for a large percentage of serious spinal injuries. Or the onset of back pain can be sudden and inexplicable. My own pinched spinal nerve occurred mysteriously at the end of a three-day meeting at which experts had discussed program, planning, and budgets—the subjects, I always felt reproachfully, perhaps contributing as much to the spine's rebellion as the three days of immobility. Trouble may start with intermittent warnings of pain that can become chronic if not treated early by corrective exercises, posture changes, bracing, even adjustments in the thickness of the soles of shoes to compensate for the slight difference in leg lengths common to most of us. "Think back" becomes a daily reminder and what Dr. Finneson calls "defensive low-back living" a necessary life-style.

Psychiatrists speculate that back pain may be a symbolic way for expressing an emotional load too heavy for some people to bear. Or it may be a physical device for relieving guilt feelings by suffering. The "bad back" is sometimes a convenient excuse for avoiding sex. In many occupations, back problems are an inherent risk. Especially vulnerable are dentists, surgeons, assembly line workers, clerks, hairdressers, and others who every day spend hours on their feet.

When chronic back pain sufferers go to hospitals for traction, bed rest, ultrasound, bracing, or surgery, they encounter in staff members a peculiar, ingrained disparagement: In disease echelons, low back pain is the nadir. Hospital staff members "do not view such patients as highly desirable," Carolyn L. Wiener discovered in her study[4] of patients with low back pain in the orthopedic ward of a large metropolitan hospital. During three months of observation, she interviewed patients, nurses on all three shifts, physicians, and physiotherapists.

Though many of the patients had verifiable problems —spinal fusions that did not "take," renewed pressure on nerves, herniated disks, or permanent damage to nerve roots—many hospital staff members were not convinced that the pain was "real," suspecting it to be largely psychogenic. (As René Leriche said, "There is only one pain that is easy to bear and that is the pain of others.") In the hospital, patients and staff square off for what must be the most unevenly matched example of gamesmanship. The staff has unwritten "rules" about appropriate pain behavior which they expect patients to abide by. The trouble is that they do not tell the patients what the rules are.

Without knowing about the patients' outside circumstances, their worries about family, job, money, and health, or the history of previous suffering and how they have coped with it, all the myriad influences that affect pain perception, the staff evaluates pain according to their notions of its nature and severity. The hidden rules also cover acceptable pain behavior. It is acceptable, for instance, for a patient to show signs of pain "ideally, three to four hours after medication—but during the interval, he is supposed to endure his pain." The staff favors "teeth gritters" and the "silent endurers," applying their own set of personal ethical values to the patient's condition, disregarding the fact that prolonged suffering and severe depression may have devitalized patients and depleted their store of stoicism.

Psychological and social clues to the "whole person" are not included in the patient's medical records, Mrs. Wiener reports:

> This dearth of information may be because psychological information is not viewed as crucial to care, and staff accountability is primarily procedural: that is, nurses are responsible for an array of treatments and procedures and are held accountable for not carrying them out, but there is no accountability for failure to listen, to understand, or to provide comfort care for the patient.
>
> It has been suggested that a specific pain profile might be drawn up upon the patient's admission, containing questions, for example, on home and hospital [pain] management. Did you have a special routine pattern at home for handling your pain? What has helped your pain in previous hospitalizations—medication, certain behavior? Is there anything in particular you would like us to know about your pain situation—any special ways of dealing with it?

Without such information, nurses put together bits and pieces about the patient's pain behavior based on their observations, their conclusions often reached when "the patient is in distress, crying, or begging for relief." This method of assessment results in the stereotyping of patients as chrons, clock watchers, malingerers, manipulators, and if they beg too often for pain relievers, addicts.

> In these days of people power, it is noteworthy that hospitals are not at all organized around patient autonomy

and patient rights. . . . Patients may make requests, but power and authority are weighted in favor of the staff. When a patient makes claims on his own behalf or appears too knowledgeable, staff members may read this as a sign that they are losing control over him. Seen as stepping on the exclusive domain of the staff, such patients are often stereotyped as manipulators, with the result that both patient and staff begin to think of themselves in an adversary relationship.

Perhaps second to his pain, the hospitalized patient's worst problem is that there is no one person who is his advocate and to whom he can address his need for pain relief. He is obliged to appeal to a variety of health-care persons responsible for aspects of his treatment and care who have the advantage over him of getting together at staff meetings and sharing their impressions of him, including their assessment of his suffering.

Mrs. Wiener's study is one of three on pain management in hospitals conducted under the direction of Dr. Anselm Strauss, professor of sociology at the University of California of San Francisco, and funded by the Division of Nursing of the Department of Health, Education, and Welfare. Reports of these studies, published in *Nursing Outlook*,[5] expose the consequences in human distress caused by the diffused responsibility in hospitals for pain management and by capricious pain assessment.

Staff assessment of pain is based on subjective judgments, influenced considerably by cultural, ethical, religious, and professional prejudices. This personalized judgment is tolerated despite the fact that the foremost pain research scientists, after years of investigation, have yet to come up with an objective, reliable means for assessing the nature and degree of pain in others. In his studies of pain patients, Dr. Ronald Melzack, a world-recognized authority on pain mechanisms and behavior,

approximates an assessment of pain by using an elaborate combination of patients' subjective assessments—
selecting from a list of 100 terms those that describe
their pain at a certain time—and extensive psychological tests, observation, and interviews conducted by psychologists and specially trained nurses. How, then, can
nurses with none of these measuring techniques at their
command assess the pain of people they scarcely know,
to say nothing of their lack of understanding about the
ineffably complex subject of pain itself? There is no
more validity for this sort of staff assessment than using
a patient's horoscope as the basis for pain treatment.

The blame, though, cannot be placed squarely on
nurses. To fault them is like criticizing the waiter for
middling food when the problem is in the kitchen—the
chef. It is the physicians who are responsible for managing chronic pain of their hospitalized patients. While
intellectually fiercely possessive of that responsibility,
they in fact abrogate it to the hospital staff. Pain control
is incidental to treatment in the hospital. The physician's
defense, that his job is to cure, narrowly defines his role
as healer.

In the medical literature, most of the articles on ameliorating chronic pain are by and for nurses. Doctors, in
their journals or on platforms at medical meetings, have
yet to address themselves to the need for giving chronic
pain management a priority in the hospital treatment
protocol, nor have they acknowledged that chronic pain
management is a new specialty, using psychological and
medical techniques quite different from those applied
to controlling acute pain.

In modern chronic pain control, opiates and surgery,
the two traditional methods, are being supplanted or
modified. Pain specialists rely far less on opiates and

surgery than do private practitioners. New treatment methods such as operant conditioning and biofeedback require active mental participation and exertion of the will, difficult to obtain if patients are dulled by drugs. Drastic surgical procedures, like cutting nerves, once the only option for people with intractable pain, are now in the same category surgery was before the discovery of anesthesia—a last resort. Many neurosurgical operations, especially those performed on the spine, have not only failed to bring permanent relief from pain, but have done lasting damage to patients.

Since the 1960s, treatment options for pain control have proliferated. Some of the methods now used are:

- Acupuncture
- Analgesics
- Autogenic training
- Biofeedback
- Chemonucleolysis
- Diet
- Dorsal column stimulators
- Exercise
- Facet nerve fulgeration
- Faith healing
- Hot and cold treatments
- Hypnosis
- Intensive family therapy
- Massage
- Operant conditioning
- Psychiatric counseling
- Psychotherapy
- Selective nerve blocks
- Self-help group therapy
- Steroids
- Surgery

· Transcutaneous nerve stimulation
· Transcendental meditation
· Ultrasonic therapy

An indirect form of pain therapy is patient participation in research studies. Subjects suffering from chronic pain become objects of special attention from the research team. Some behavioral tests require a fair amount of concentration that shifts the focus from physical discomfort to an assessment of personality traits, a new experience for many patients. The research-treatment team enters into an informal contractual agreement with the patients, who are expected to take some responsibility in their treatment program.

Dr. Wilbert E. Fordyce, professor of clinical psychology at the University of Washington, says that people who have better things to do don't hurt so much. Perhaps, he concedes, they actually hurt as much, but what counts is that they can assign to pain a lesser priority in their scheme of things. Dr. Fordyce is credited with pioneering the application of "operant conditioning" to pain behavior. Operant conditioning was developed by behavioral scientists in animal behavior studies, using the principle of rewards for learning. In their laboratory experiments, psychologists trained monkeys, pigeons, and other creatures to push the right buttons to get the reward of their favorite food. In his rehabilitation center at the University of Washington, Dr. Fordyce adapts this learning-reward principle to chronic pain patients. Those who make an effort to walk despite discomfort, who do things for themselves, and who surpass treatment goals are rewarded with praise and attention. Patients who have used their pain as a psychological weapon, who make no effort, who subtly sabotage their treatment program are ignored. Generally, shamed by the progress of more severely handicapped patients, and unhappy about losing the respect of the staff, those patients pull themselves together and make an effort.

The behavioral scientists in the rehabilitation program are fully aware that pain of psychological origin—"wounds of the spirit"—can hurt as much as a bad burn or a severe cramp in the leg. What Dr. Fordyce and his associates try to do is to get at the root of the psychological problem while treating the pain itself.

"People can learn to hurt and learn not to hurt," Dr. Fordyce says. The original cause of the pain may have been long since corrected, yet, "the pain bell continues to ring." In the retraining process, medication is not given on demand, but at fixed intervals, regardless of how the patient feels. The analgesic is mixed in a pleasant-tasting syrup, the amount of the analgesic systematically reduced as the patient's dependence on it and need for it diminish.

After an assessment of the patient's ability to perform, exercises are prescribed that conform to a reasonable quota of effort slightly below the patient's capability, thus encouraging him or her by success to make an effort to exceed the quota. Therapeutic activities designed to counteract the disability help in turn in the management of the pain. People who have used canes for years are encouraged and trained to walk without them. Patients who have developed posture distortions to favor pain take special exercises to help them sit and walk normally.

It doesn't help much to change a patient's behavior patterns unless there are changes in the behavior of those around him. By being oversolicitous, or sanctifying the suffering person, or putting up with tantrums, families inadvertently reinforce pain behavior. Only those patients whose families agree to reinforce the principles of the program are accepted at Dr. Fordyce's center.

Some key member of the family, usually a spouse, or, if the patient is unmarried, a boy friend or girl friend, is given special training in the new roles, usually at one or two sessions a week. Dr. Fordyce considers the training of spouses an integral component of treatment, without which the whole effort may be nullified. Instead of over-protecting the sufferer, families are cautioned against doing things for a person he could well do for himself with some effort, or even slight discomfort. The success of the treatment depends on how well the patient continues to practice what he has learned in the pain rehabilitation center and on the support he gets from his family.[6]

Another innovation in pain control is biofeedback, which has been described by one of its pioneers, Dr. Barbara B. Brown,[7] as "a tuning-in to the interior self," the interior world taking directions from the mind, rediscovering the will and its power. That we can control the body's inner workings and responses is by no means a new discovery—people have allowed themselves to be buried alive for days, have walked on fiery coals, and slept on sharp pointed nails. But scientific theories about the inner mechanisms of control and the machines that visualize internal changes are products of the electronic age. Biofeedback trains people to relax and at the same time to control bodily functions they had considered automatic and uncontrollable, like heart rate and blood flow. It is especially effective for types of pain related to tension, headaches, muscle spasms, low back pain, and arthritic flare-ups.

In this kind of therapy, the person sits comfortably in a chair or lies on a bed. Electrodes attached to the skin by small rubber cups extend to a machine that monitors the internal functions he is trying to control, recording the results on a screen or meter. With training and intense concentration, a person can reduce painful muscular tension, control heartbeat rate, skin temperature, and peripheral blood flow. Using whatever means he chooses—thinking quiet thoughts, visualizing pleasant scenes—the person relaxes and the machine tells him how well he is doing. Once the control skills are mastered, a person can call upon them at will without being attached to a machine. The technique develops self-reliance and confidence and in many cases reduces the need for analgesics.

A widely used pain control mechanism is the transcutaneous nerve stimulator developed by Dr. C. Norman Shealy in 1960. This device controls pain from the surface of the skin by stimulating nerves involved in the pain process, using the principle of counterstimulation. Easily carried in a pocket, the small transistorized generator has twin electrodes that, when pain attacks, are placed on the skin either in the pain area or over major nerve pathways. Electrical pulses pass through the skin, their strength, pulse rate, and duration adjusted by a dial. As a method of pain treatment approved by Medicare, costs of the device can be reimbursed by the government. The devices, sold commercially by many firms, are used for acute and chronic pain. They can be applied temporarily for relief or strapped in place and worn continually. Though they give prompt relief for chronic pain, they do not cure it, but by alleviating it, make it more tolerable. Used in conjunction with other types of pain treatment, this device helps patients loosen their clutch on analgesic drugs not only because of the relief, but because they are released from the fear that without drugs nothing can help them.

Though physicians deride it and science gives it no

place, faith healing is an essential element in medicine. At least 80 percent of all healing is a matter of faith. How many cures would a doctor bring about if he did not believe in his powers to cure and if the patient did not share that belief? Surgeons know the risk they take when they operate on a patient who has no faith in the surgeon's ability to help him, who is convinced he will die on the operating table. Experienced surgeons refuse in many instances to operate on such doubting patients.

Does the patient know what is in those two-color pills he takes every day and how they work inside him? Yet, he takes them faithfully every day. Without faith there would be no medical care. Among many health practitioners there has been a resurgence of interest in the ancient art of faith healing, the "laying on of hands." Dr. Dolores Kreiger, professor of nursing at New York University, has introduced the technique in hospitals and schools of nursing throughout the country. She calls her method "therapeutic touch," a method that can be taught, a way of transmitting bodily energy to a person whose illness or pain has reduced his own bodily energy.

Inherent in this system is transmitting not only energy, but a strong sense of caring for the person and in the process helping restore the energy he needs to restore himself. Studies show that changes take place in metabolism and in enzyme systems during this transfer of energy. Dr. Kreiger does not use the term "laying on of hands," for in her therapeutic touch method she does not touch a person, but holds her hands an inch or so away from the patient. The healer creates a field of energy through the hands that induces chemical changes in the body. Dr. Kreiger has taught this method to 3,000 nurses, therapists, physicians, and medical students.

This renewal of an ancient art is one manifestation of

disillusion with modern medicine, its impersonality and mechanization. The World Health Organization in 1977 announced that it was turning to unorthodox methods of healing, including faith healing, to achieve its goals of improving world health. And in America, younger health practitioners are far less skeptical about the powers of folk medicine than most of their elders.

Svengali, the mesmerist in the novel *Trilby*, gave hypnosis such a bad name it is only now recovering. Without fanfare, some dentists have used hypnosis successfully for decades with patients whose heart conditions or other medical problems make the use of anesthetics too risky. The current success of hypnosis in pain control is restoring its reputation with the public and the medical profession. When Dr. Harold J. Wain, a medical psychologist and director of the Psychiatry Liaison and Consultation Service at Walter Reed Army Medical Center in Washington, D.C., introduced hypnosis as a treatment method at the center's pain clinic, his colleagues were not enthusiastic. But, when patients demonstrated that hypnosis enabled them to cut down on pain medication and avoid surgery, he established hypnosis as a bona fide method of pain control. It is now part of the training for psychiatric residents and psychology interns at the Army Medical Center.

Success with this method, says Dr. Wain, depends largely on the patient's motivation, his "gift" for hypnosis, and the strategy the doctor uses. Exploding the myth that the best subjects for hypnosis are the gullible or the naïve, he says that a well-disciplined mind responds best to hypnosis. Candidates for this type of pain treatment are first screened by what is called the Hypnotic Induction Profile and by clinical interviews.

"In a busy medical center," Dr. Wain says, "we have to decide which patients will most benefit from hypnosis and then to base our treatment strategy on what we learn in our test and interviews with a patient. For instance, I ask patients what has worked for them in reducing their pain, what exacerbates it, their recreational interests, how they relax, and so on. Their responses determine some of the strategies we use while they are in a trance state. We help them reinterpret the meaning pain has for them. We help them decrease their anxiety and their anticipation of pain, as well as insulate themselves from discomfort. The very least hypnosis does is to reduce anxiety and that in itself reduces pain."

Hypnosis, for some, cuts through quickly to underlying psychological problems. But in some instances there may not *be* a deep psychological problem. If psychological problems do exist, however, the less severe they are, the more effective the hypnosis. "Hypnosis helps patients deal with pain that has a physical basis. Athletes," says Dr. Wain, "do that all the time, continuing to play despite severe physical injury. That's a form of auto-hypnosis. In fact, one of our goals is to teach every patient auto-hypnosis. Our post-hypnotic suggestions reinforce a sense of feeling better and give them a sense of mastery over their symptoms. Using hypnosis to teach patients pain control and self-reliance makes them more independent and more responsible for their own comfort. In some instances, when patients have difficulty with auto-hypnosis, possibly for some psychological reasons, we give them tape recordings as a back-up, but we prefer that they be as self-reliant as possible. Some patients need their pain for psychological reasons. When that is evident, the patient keeps the pain, but by hypnosis the intensity of it can be modified so they can cope with it without unnecessary medical aid that might have complications."[8]

An organized method of pain management is the pain

clinic. In 1975 when I was doing research for this book, there was no list of pain clinics in the United States. Two years later the American Society of Anesthesiologists published the first directory,[9] listing 330 pain clinics, their locations, types of pain treated, medical specialties of the staffs, and methods of treatment.

Costs at pain clinics vary. Those in Veterans Administrative hospitals are usually based on ability to pay. At university hospital pain clinics, a treatment program of several months may cost $5,000 or more. Pain clinics within hospitals charge regular hospital rates, with extra charges for certain procedures. Treatment in outpatient clinics is generally less expensive. Some clinics treat only inpatients, others only outpatients, and some both types. A few clinics specialize in one type of pain, such as headaches or backaches. The range of treatment methods depends on the specialists either on the clinic staff or those available from hospital departments.

Though the incidence of chronic pain, research advances, and new treatment methods account for much of the phenomenal growth of these clinics, a significant boost came from the authority for Medicare reimbursement for treatment costs. The goal of Medicare support, according to the official guidelines, "is to give the patient tools to manage and control his pain and thereby improve his ability to function independently." The guidelines spell out the types of treatment that would be given, responsibilities of nurses, and the supervisory role of physicians. Though the treatment programs approved for Medicare payment are primarily hospital based, the regulations open the door for reimbursement for outpatient treatment.

Physicians differ about what an ideal pain clinic should be. Should it be in a hospital or free-standing? Should it serve inpatients or outpatients, or both? Should it specialize in one type of pain? Is it necessary that there be a multidisciplinary staff?

Dr. Benjamin Kripke, professor and associate chairman, Boston University School of Medicine, and clinical director of anesthesia at the University Hospital, favors what he calls "mini pain centers" under hospital aegis. An integral part of the clinic's pain management program should be a home care program. Among services available to the mini centers from the hospital staff would be those given by anesthesiologists, neurologists, internists, rheumatologists, oncologists, psychiatrists, nurses, and therapists.

In Dr. Kripke's view, the specialists should not be full-time members of the clinic staff. One reason is that pain control practice offers small financial returns for the private practitioner, about one-fifth of what an anesthesiologist makes in his field. Physicians, Dr. Kripke said in an interview, cannot afford to devote themselves entirely to pain control practice even with "third-party" (insurance) payments. But by drawing on hospital staff as needed, mini pain centers could be self-supporting.

Dr. Kripke sees the progression of pain management beginning with treating the physical cause of it. If primary care does not cure the pain, the private physician refers the patient to a group of pain specialists, while becoming a member of the consulting group, in that way keeping his ties with the patient. Pain specialists, besides their medical expertise, need the temperament for long-term relationships with patients, a background in psychology, and the ability to talk informally with patients.

The present demand for pain treatment far exceeds the resources of facilities and physicians and medical assistants trained in pain management. All pain clinics have waiting lists. The University of Illinois Medical Center in Chicago, following a series of television programs on a nonsurgical procedure for treating slipped disks, was so overwhelmed by the number of inquiries about the treatment that Dr. Alon P. Winnie, head of the anesthesiology department, had to resort to a form letter for replies. In it, he explained the physiology of a slipped disk, the traditional treatment, and the injection therapy used at the university's pain clinic. He went a step further by giving each inquirer the names and addresses of doctors in the inquirer's vicinity who use the same therapy, which has had a success rate of 80 to 90 percent in patients who have never had disk surgery, in other words, "virgin backs."

At most pain clinics, the first appraisal of a patient includes a physical and psychological examination. These tests and personal interviews tell the psychologists something about the "whole person" and give a clue to how well the person is likely to respond to treatment. Understandably, all pain clinics use screening methods to spare themselves costly waste of staff time and effort on patients who make a career of doctor shopping or those whose payoffs from pain, financial or psychological, are likely to undermine their motivation after they get into the program.

At the Pain Center directed by Dr. Bonica at the University of Washington, the first to use the multidisciplinary approach to the diagnosis and treatment of pain of unknown origin, each patient is assigned a medical manager, a physician who is in charge of the patient from the time he or she is admitted until he or she leaves. After being evaluated by specialists from several disciplines, the patient appears with his or her medical manager before the team. The problem is presented, and the patient answers questions from the psychologist, social worker, neurosurgeon, and other members of the team. The patient then leaves the room and the team members discuss the patient's personality, the nature and possible causes of the pain, and conditions that may be contributing to the pain, such as an unhappy marriage, heavy debts, or rejection by children. The team then decides on a treatment program geared to that person's situation.

At the pain clinic of the Scripps Clinic Medical Institutions in La Jolla, California, Dr. Richard Sternbach developed a battery of questions as guides for treatment. The question that usually brings patients up short is: How would you live if you got rid of the pain? Most people with chronic pain have been so intent on their suffering and their desire to get rid of it that they haven't thought much about the alternatives. Suddenly, they are confronted by the options. What would be the financial losses or gains? Could they get jobs that would bring them in as much or more than disability payments? What changes would occur in their role in the family? Would they gain new respect or lose a pampered position? If a patient has used chronic pain as an excuse for avoiding social life, would he or she make the effort to rejoin the world? How would the person compensate for the loss of attention from family, friends, and physicians? Is the role of a suffering person too satisfying to relinquish?

Answers to those and other disconcerting questions indicate whether a patient is ready for treatment. Based on his experience with hundreds of pain patients, Dr. Sternbach has come up with these general guidelines[10] for predicting the chances of success or failure in pain treatment:

- Married with family to support—good
- Formerly married but living alone—not so good
- Satisfying sexual life before onset of pain—good

- Unsatisfying sexual life before onset of pain—not so good
- Continuing to work despite pain—good
- Has not worked for some time—not so good
- Supported by disability, unemployment, or welfare benefits—very poor
- Manages without using prescribed analgesics—good
- Medically dependent on narcotics—can be helped
- Immediately took to drugs and persisted in their use—poor

The treatment program in the San Diego Veterans Administration Hospital pain ward, established by Dr. Sternbach, includes daily group therapy sessions, attended by the pain patients, nurses, and the psychologist. Patients talk about their anxieties and the type and degree of their pain. Members of the staff and other patients comment on each patient's pain problem. "One of the benefits of these sessions," says Dr. Sternbach in his book, *Pain Patients*, "is that the patients quickly realize that they are not alone, that others have been struggling and suffering and manipulating as they have, and that there is understanding of what they have been through. This seems to make for an *esprit de corps* which provides a setting in which patients feel more comfortable asking whether, for example, their low-back pain will lead to paralysis, or if they have cancer, and similar fears which they previously felt too inhibited to express."

Group discussion also enables patients to realize how they use their pain for payoffs in sympathy, narcotics, financial compensation, or admiration for bravery, payoffs usually not sought consciously. When a patient's pain game is described to him by other patients who have played similar games, Dr. Sternbach says, he is more inclined to accept it and to analyze his behavior.

"This is more effective than when feedback is provided by the staff. Patients may deceive themselves and the staff, but they cannot long deceive other patients with whom they are living, and feedback from the others, given supportively, soon stops the game playing."

At the Boston Pain Unit directed by Dr. Gerald M. Aronoff, who specializes in stress and behavioral medicine, patients are urged to take more responsibility for their own health instead of passively relinquishing the care to others. Patients at this unit are not only responsible for aspects of their own care, but for helping each other. They are not treated as sore backs, legs, or arms, but as whole people, important units in a family and their community.

Treatment includes physical therapy, biofeedback, hypnosis, nerve stimulation as well as conventional pain medications and other therapies. A main emphasis is on helping the patient change his attitudes toward his pain. The average patient is in his late forties, has had three unsuccessful operations, and has not improved under conventional treatment. Patients are encouraged to talk about their experiences, to vent repressed anger and frustrations induced by hated bosses, or nagging wives, or intolerable brothers. In some of these patients, depression, always present to an extent in chronic pain, has been exacerbated by the negative attitude of their personal physicians. One woman patient who had suggested to her doctor that physical therapy might help her was told abruptly that she was too old. Nevertheless, she applied for admission to the rehabilitation pain unit, was accepted, and improved by changing her perspective on the pain and by elevating her self-respect.

Careful selection and good pain management, says Dr. Aronoff, do not always ensure success. A patient on workmen's compensation who had had a series of back operations went through the treatment and felt fine. But after leaving the unit, he could not cope with the trials of job hunting. The lure of the assured compensation check was so strong that he found a doctor willing to certify him as totally disabled.

"The goal of medicine and insurance companies," says Dr. Aronoff, "is to get people back to work. Here at the pain unit, our goals are broader. We want patients to get back to work too, but we want them to be glad to get up in the morning, to feel like smiling, not only with restored or improved functions, but no longer willing to spend their days in bed, sleeping hours away, drugged by medication. We select our patients carefully for the same reasons other pain clinics do, to prevent wasted services, efforts, and money on drop-outs, but there's another reason. We don't want these people, regardless of what pain gains they are protecting, to suffer one more failure, one more injury to an already damaged self-image. But our selection process does not exclude many whose medical histories might indicate certain failure. We had one patient who had had 26 unsuccessful operations, not exactly a likely candidate for success. But in the supportive atmosphere of the unit and with first-rate medical treatment, this man made surprising headway in managing his pain and in coping with the psychological problems that had contributed to his condition."

For people looking for pain clinics there is the directory published by the American Association of Anesthesiologists, but nothing yet to help in selecting a clinic. Some considerations to be taken into account are:

· The location of the clinic (important from a convenience standpoint, but nearness may not be the best criterion)

- Types of pain treated
- Types of treatment
- Specialties represented on the staff or available to the clinic from an affiliated hospital or medical center
- Criteria for admitting patients (Some pain clinics do not take patients who are involved in pending suits for injuries that have caused chronic pain. Other clinics exclude people on disability compensation, and some have age limits.)
- Procedure for admission (whether a referral is required from a physician or the clinic considers application directly from a possible patient)
- Average length of treatment
- Inpatients only—outpatients only—or both
- Average cost of treatment
- Eligibility for Medicare reimbursement
- Home-care program
- Follow-up program
- Is there a waiting list of patients?
- Are patients with terminal cancer, arthritis, or diabetes accepted?
- Does the clinic have a tie-in with a medical and nursing teaching institution?
- Does the clinic conduct research? (If so, and patients are subjects in research projects, what is the system for protecting them?)

Pain clinics have been called medicine's growth industry. They are a boon to harassed physicians who now have a place to which they can refer patients they can no longer help. And for the chronic pain sufferers, they are a refuge where they are taken care of by skilled professionals who have chosen pain management because it is a new, challenging, and gratifying specialty.

As more families are being bankrupted by hospital and nursing-home care, home care becomes a sensible alternative. Voluntary agencies and some commercial companies provide medical and home-management services. Practical nurses are being trained in taking care of patients who have acute and chronic pain. Linda D. Winslow, instructor at the Shepard Gill School of Practical Nursing in Boston, prepared guidelines for practical nurses that could be applied by members of any family that has the home care of someone suffering from prolonged pain. The emphasis is on comfort and care, making a comfortable bed, administering a bath, giving frequent back care, listening with an inner ear for unspoken anxieties. Part of "sensory comfort" is shutting out excessive noise, adjusting disturbing light, or keeping the room free of clutter. "The practical nurse," says Linda Winslow, "learns how to assess her own attitudes toward pain and people who have it, to uncover hidden prejudices against those who suffer and resentment over manifestations of it."[11]

Unless the disease state warrants it, hospitalization for chronic pain is an excessive solution for the problem. In hospice programs, people with severe pain are kept comfortable at home as long as possible, sometimes for years. Pain medication is administered on a regular schedule and in doses that keep the person alert, but free of pain. Nutritious meals are part of pain management at home. The better a person's physical condition, the better he or she can cope with pain. As Dr. Richard Lamerton, director of St. Joseph's Hospice in London, puts it, the aim of home care is to keep a person comfortable and spare him or her the horrors of hospitalization, afflicted by "last minute operations, tubes in every orifice, dramatic and violent resuscitations; friends and relatives kept at bay by visiting hours and the hospital staff by their busyness."

A pain reliever you'll not find listed in any physician's handbook, but the most ancient of all, is the friendly visit. Amusing talk, a ration or two of titillating gossip, a classmate's account of the school day, the latest news from the office political front, spiritual comfort and a laugh or two with a young chaplain, the silent exchange between two people holding hands, each in its own way the diversion of good company that diminishes the awareness of pain and discomfort. A visit to the sick and suffering is "twice blessed," giving an inner satisfaction to the visitor and relieving pain and tedium for the visited.

But there is an art to it. Kathryn Himmelsbach, as a social worker who has observed the interactions of hundreds of visitors and patients in the cancer unit of the National Institutes of Health Clinical Center, says that a visit to the suffering is a way of saying "Someone cares about you," a reaffirmation that the person is important, worth caring about. That's why a visit to someone confined to a hospital, a nursing home, or his or her own home takes on a significance those of us who are well and able to get about cannot fully comprehend.

Most people are uneasy about visiting patients who are very ill or in severe pain. Mrs. Himmelsbach attributes that feeling to our fear that it might happen to us, a reminder of our own vulnerability. "For this reason," she says, "there are people who cannot transcend their own self-consciousness and look at the visit from the viewpoint of the patient."

Self-conscious visitors are quite apt to breeze into a sick room and, scarcely glancing at the patient, tell him, "My, how well you look!" The patient knows he looks ghastly. He's sick and may be hurting very badly. "It's not at all helpful to play games with that kind of reality," Mrs. Himmelsbach says. "Nor is it helpful to try to identify with the sufferer by going into a tirade about the injustice of his suffering. Or questioning how a loving God of the Sunday school picture books could suddenly strike a hammer blow against such a saintly person. Patients have difficulties enough coming to terms with their own feelings of doubt and guilt without assistance from an overwrought visitor."

Visits would be more successful if visitors appreciated the impact of the visit on the patient. It is an event. The visitor who is ill at ease, who is far more aware of his own reactions to the sights, sounds, and smells than to what his visit signifies to the sick person, nullifies his own good intentions. Awkward, stiff visits are trying experiences for everyone, but they can be transformed into gratifying ones.

Mrs. Himmelsbach gives the three main elements in the successful visit: body language, tone of voice, and control of the visit. A visitor should move close to the patient, should touch him. Depending on the relationship, the touch may be a warm, friendly handshake or an affectionate embrace. "Instead of standing at a distance, as if poised for flight, the visitor should sit down. And not on the edge of the chair."

The hospital setting erects physical and psychological barriers to satisfactory conversation. The patient is at a decided disadvantage, first, because he is in discomfort and then, too, he is not on his own turf, not in charge of anything, not even of his own body. "Whatever a visitor can do to restore even a small sense of control to the patient helps restore a sense of self esteem."

There are times and circumstances when there is great solace in the silence that flows between two people when there is love and understanding. "And merely holding a patient's hand can be wonderfully comforting. Even the tone of voice influences the patient and the visit itself. Some visitors, including members of the family, speak as if they were in a mortuary. Acting in a totally unnatural way merely increases the tension."

Visiting someone who is ill at home is usually much less strained than at the hospital or nursing home. A chronically ill person at home needs the stimulation of people; television is not enough, its level of stimulation rarely high enough to raise the pain threshold. A living, breathing, talking person can work wonders.

It takes great poise and self-discipline to visit someone who is obviously in severe pain, whose pallor and facial expressions, despite valiant efforts of control, betray the person's discomfort. Mrs. Himmelsbach advises visitors not to ignore such manifestations as though they were not taking place or were somehow shameful. "Many cancer patients are proud of the way they cope with their pain. It's like telling someone about an arduous experience we've handled well. We expect some acknowledgment, a psychological stroke. In the circumscribed world of the cancer patient, whether in the hospital or home, the struggle to exert some personal control over pain, not depending entirely on medication, can be heroic. It would be mean-spirited indeed not to acknowledge that effort."

Ill-at-ease visitors sometimes feel impelled to make themselves useful by fixing pillows, smoothing out sheets, rearranging things on the bedside table. Fussing around can irritate a patient and, like anxiety, irritation increases sensitivity to pain. The anxious, restless visitor may do more harm than good and might do better by sending flowers.

Gauging the length of the visit requires intuition, sensitivity, and finesse. The visit should not be sandwiched in between a tight schedule of parking meter tyranny, hair appointments, meetings, or flight departures. Clock watching by a visitor is bad manners. Patient watching, on the other hand, is essential to a mutually satisfying visit. Even though a patient may be visibly tired and suffering, he may dread being left alone with his pain and may cling to the visit as to a life preserver. This is the moment the visitor's intuition must guide him. If he decides to go, he should do so with finesse, his leave-taking conveying warmth and genuine feeling even though it is expressed casually. And, as in the beginning of the visit, the importance of physical contact, the handclasp, a hug, a kiss, even stroking the skin on the back of a hand.

No one, says Mrs. Himmelsbach, should visit a person he hates. If for compelling social or business reasons, some acknowledgment of an ailing enemy is necessary, send a card or an impersonal plant.

7 | "Suffer little children ..."

"Children don't have chronic pain. They either quickly recover or they die."

This flat, dismissive statement, made to me at the outset of my research for this book, typifies the brand of denial which pervades the medical profession, a refusal to recognize the suffering by children as if it were a distraction from the primary business of curing. In the months that followed the pronouncement of that pediatrician, from talks with physicians, nurses, public health administrators, clergymen, scientists, psychologists, and therapists, a quite different picture emerged. They were ready enough to discuss chronic pain in adults, but when my questions veered toward prolonged suffering in sick and injured children, suddenly there was a reticence, a backing off, the surreptitious closing of doors. It seemed that there was about this subject an unconscious conspiracy of denial.

Among physicians this denial, more perhaps a disregard, was especially marked. Neither callous nor cruel, their attitude was more a turning away from a situation they felt helpless to control. It was as if, intent on curing, exerting to the utmost their skills, conscientiously doing their jobs as healers, they could not allow themselves to be deflected from their main purpose even by ac-

139

knowledging the pain they caused or the suffering inherent in a disease, a treatment procedure, or an injury. Most doctors I asked about pain control in children said the available analgesics were adequate or they suggested I interview the hospital psychiatrist.

"Drawing out the marrow of the bones of leukemic children really isn't such a painful procedure," an oncologist told me. "I've had it done to me when I was a hospital resident. We used to practice the technique on each other, hitting the right spot on the cusp of the hip bone, inserting the needle, then drawing out some marrow with a syringe. Oh, there was a faintly unpleasant sensation, but it wasn't especially painful. I don't think it bothers the children very much."

The doctor who made that statement was a big, healthy man. He and his fellow residents were practicing a technique, not undergoing a diagnostic test on the progress of a deadly disease. Nor were they faced with the prospect of bone punctures and marrow aspirations twice or three times a week during intensive therapy when the progress of anticancer drugs is closely monitored in laboratory tests of the marrow.

Bone marrow is the organ that manufactures the normal blood cells, red and white cells, the latter the body's defenders against harmful invaders. In leukemia, something goes wrong with this manufacturing process. Instead of producing normal ones, defective white cells are manufactured, proliferating wildly and preventing the growth of normal red and white cells. Leukemic cells may get into the bloodstream and circulate throughout the body, damaging the liver, spleen, lymph nodes, or other organs. This disease, once fatal within a few months, now has a survival rate of five or more years for 50 percent of children treated with anticancer drugs.

Leukemia itself in its early stages is not painful, but

the diagnostic and treatment methods are. During the intensive treatment phase, blood is drawn from the fingers three or four times a week, hip and breastbones are punctured and the marrow drawn out, and needles are inserted in veins for the continuous infusion of anticancer drugs into the system. These drugs cause the hair to fall out, nausea, mouth and stomach ulcers, constipation, wobbly legs, rashes, nightmares, irritability, and changes in the personality. Each bone marrow aspiration may mean reprieve or a renewed massive onslaught of the horrendous anticancer drugs.

Their bodies depleted by the disease and drugs, the children experience almost insupportable anxiety. In some hospitals where no medication is given the children to reduce anxiety, drawing out the marrow becomes a painful and terrifying procedure. It is often necessary for several attendants to restrain a screaming, thrashing child. Wild, chaotic scenes take place, infuriating to a doctor trying to push a needle into the bone and drawing out the marrow without breaking the needle, exasperating to the nurse who is supposed to maintain a calm atmosphere, and unforgettable to the child. Quite a different scene from that in which several young, healthy hospital residents practice on each other, exchanging gibes and good-natured insults when clumsy fingers miss the mark. Years later, it did not seem unrealistic to one of those residents who has experienced one bone aspiration to compare it to that of a very sick child, frightened and apprehensive, who, during a long period of intensive treatment, may have a hip or breastbone pierced two or three times a week and feel, as the marrow is drawn out, the tearing of tiny, sensitive nerve endings.

And how do the children themselves, even the stoical ones, perceive this procedure? They call the day marrow is to be drawn out "'Bone Day," anticipated with fear and near-panic. It is the time they most want their mothers to be with them or a trusted member of the hospital staff, someone to be near them, to hold their hands, and stroke their foreheads. Stoical as many are during the procedure, their true feelings show up later in their childlike drawings.

No one knows better than Susan Castelluccio, art therapist who works with hospitalized children, what "Bone Day" means to the children. She has seen in its aftermath the drawings of planes crashing in flames, huge spears aimed at a stick-figure child, helplessly awaiting the attack. Small children are rarely articulate about their suffering from bone marrow aspirations, or the succession of finger stickings to draw blood samples, or the nausea from the drugs, or the discomfort of needles stuck in their veins slowly feeding the powerful anticancer drugs into their systems. But at their bedsides or in the special playrooms where the children draw pictures with colored crayons or paints, Susan Castelluccio learns how the children feel about pain.

Seated beside a child, she gets him or her to tell what the drawing means. Usually simple stick figures represent the child, but some children with a flair for drawing adapt comic-strip figures. Without seeming to pattern her questions, Miss Castelluccio gradually gets the child to explain the sketch.

A 9-year-old boy, following "Bone Day," drew a picture of Snoopy, the dog in the famous comic strip, "Peanuts." Snoopy lies on his back on top of his doghouse. "Thought balloons" arise. In the top one, a flaming plane has nose-dived into the ground. Off to one side of the drawing is a small sketch of the comic strip Red Baron in his flying suit, watching the crash of the plane in Snoopy's fantasy. Explaining his drawing to the art therapist, the little boy says, "Snoopy is thinking about an airplane crash and the Red Baron is the brave flyer who survives the crash. And he isn't crying, he's just watching." "And where are you in the drawing?" Miss Castelluccio asks him. The child points to the Red Baron. On "Bone Day," he tells her, "I was as brave as the Red Baron. I didn't cry."

The frequency of bone marrow tests depends on the stage of the cancer. At the outset of the disease or in relapse, the treatment is intensive. Bone marrow may be tested several times a week. As the disease responds to the powerful chemical medication, bone marrow may be tested once a month. In prolonged remission, maybe once in six months. Pain and discomfort are heightened by apprehension: Children know that the results of the tests determine whether they are getting better. And getting better means going home.

Local anesthetic on the skin above the bone area dulls the pain of the needle as it punctures the skin, but no medication is given to kill the sensation of fine nerves being ripped and torn away from the bone, a sensation one child compared to having a fingernail torn off. If the needle does not pierce the bone, or breaks as sometimes happens, the doctor has to try again. The bones of young adults, harder than those of children, are especially difficult to puncture.

An adolescent girl, whose leukemia had flared up, was obliged to return to the hospital for intensive treatment. The woman doctor who did the bone marrow aspirations was not strong enough to get the needle into the breastbone without causing the girl terrible pain and distress. The woman doctor could not admit to herself that she lacked the physical strength to force the needle through the bone, no doubt feeling that physical inadequacy reflected unfavorably on her professional skill. The girl, fearful of confronting the woman doctor, finally went to a hospital administrator and told him the problem. Rather than make an issue of the matter, the administrator took no action, thereby forcing the girl to endure the torment of blundering, frustrating attempts to force the needle through the bone. To that hospital administrator, the girl's suffering was of less consequence than his maintaining smooth professional relations with a stubborn, insensitive staff physician.

When asked why pain- and anxiety-reducing medication was not given to children—and adults—undergoing this diagnostic nightmare, several physicians replied, "But it only takes ten minutes." One said, "But you wouldn't give general anesthesia for this procedure. It's too dangerous and not worth it." When pressed about alternatives to general anesthesia, the answer was usually a helpless shrug or a flash of irritation, a closing of the door.

One of the ironies that abound in the field of medicine is that the drug Laetrile, which has not been proved to be harmful and is regarded by some cancer patients as highly efficacious in arresting their disease and assuaging their pain, is banned by the Food and Drug Administration. That watchdog administration, however, sanctions the use of compounds on children and adults that are so toxic they cause hair to fall out, almost constant nausea, scales and rashes, jaundice, loss of appetite, and personality changes. These drugs are condoned in the interests of research. As a scientist working on a research project involving cancer drugs puts it: "The payoffs in cancer treatment research can be huge, so the violence of the treatment is in a sense proportionate to the benefits."

Dr. Charles B. Pratt of St. Jude Children's Research

Hospital in Memphis says there should be a more rational approach to chemotherapy in children. The enormous public pressure on doctors and scientists to come up with cures for cancer has resulted in treatment programs considered appropriate by medical practitioners that in other medical situations would be considered unethical.

"In many types of childhood cancer," Dr. Pratt said in an interview, "the treatment regimes, including overlapping cycles of as many as five to seven drugs, have been arrived at without a solid base of clinical evidence about blood levels, length of time of drug action, metabolism, and interaction among the many drugs used in the treatment. Or of the long-range effect these drugs will have on the development of the children."

Dr. Pratt considers the mental anguish engendered by the stress of the treatment equal to extreme physical pain. "It's sometimes necessary to use narcotics to relieve the mental anguish of children, even though they may not be in physical pain. But they are suffering intensely."

In St. Jude hospital, children in the final stage of painful cancer receive, with supportive fluids being fed intravenously, a dose of morphine to deaden pain. "How pain control is carried out differs from hospital to hospital and depends on the philosophy of the institution," said Dr. Pratt. "No matter how grave an illness is, it is possible to create a comforting atmosphere in a hospital, an atmosphere in which the children and their parents sense a genuine caring concern on the part of the hospital staff. At St. Jude, the children have their pain control schedules worked out to conform to their needs. The pain is anticipated, very much as in a hospice. This system of pain control greatly reduces anxiety. But we still have a long way to go in controlling pain in children. Much more attention should be given to it. Children are not small adults, but quite special physiological beings. But we force them to adjust to adult medications and types of treatment."

In cancer centers and in most cancer wards where chemotherapy, radiation, and surgical techniques are constantly undergoing testing and revision, the focus of the medical team is on arresting the wildly growing cancer cells. If a patient's hair, eyebrows, and eyelashes fall out, if he or she vomits all day, that is unfortunate, but it is not of great concern to the cancer fighters.

The patient is not a person, but a disease. The doctors' minds are on cells rather than on the human being who is the sum and the host of those cells. But the children who are the subjects of the well-intentioned treatment see themselves vividly in a different way. Susan Castelluccio interested a young black boy in drawing shortly after he was admitted to the hospital for treatment of multiple tumors. In his first drawing, he portrayed himself, not as a stick figure, but as a fully drawn child, wearing a bright blue jacket with yellow trim, dark slacks, shiny shoes, and hair, lots of it in an Afro. Sometime later the boy drew himself in a nondescript outfit of somber blacks and purples, the colors that very sick children use to portray themselves. And his head was completely bald. The last drawing in this boy's sequence was in pencil, no color whatsoever. He portrayed himself as a strange, apelike creature standing upright, the outline jagged lines. The creature is smoking a huge cigar, symbol of the manhood he knew he would never achieve. Shortly after drawing that dehumanized self, the boy died.

In their drawings, children portray death in many guises. One child drew a shark pursuing a little fish. On the shark's body were red and purple patches, indicating the places on the boy's body where tumors had been cut out. The gravely sick child explained to Miss Castelluccio that he was the shark and also the little fish pursued by the shark. A question mark above the head of the little fish indicated its worry about what was going to happen to it. Beneath the shark on the bottom of the sea, a snail goes its way, not heeding the shark or the little fish, not caring.

This sense of loneliness, of people not caring, indifferent to their suffering, is a common motif in the drawings of children who have cancer. And death rarely comes as a surprise to them. It is not unusual for them to sense it before the doctors, nurses, and their own parents know. They may confide their secret to a trusted nurse, a social worker, or an art therapist, making them promise not to tell their parents because it would make them feel sad. One motherless boy, while Susan Castelluccio was on vacation, sensing that he was dying, managed to keep alive until she returned. He had waited, he told her, so he could die in her arms, which he did the following day.

Many hospitalized children find their only emotional release through drawing and painting. Not only is it a release, but, by expressing their pain graphically, they are given a sense of control over a situation in which they are helpless. The terrible burden of suffering secretly is lessened when it can be splashed on paper in violent, bloody colors, a means of talking soundlessly about innermost feelings.

When it is most successful, this type of therapy is conducted by a therapist, an artist trained in psychology, who is accepted as a confidant by the child and is willing to stay with him or her during painful procedures. Within such a trusting relationship, the art therapist helps the child work through problems induced by illness and hospitalization, overwhelmed by strangers putting him through frightening experiences, where monster machines explore his body with invisible rays, needles puncture his fingers, bones, and spine, and surgery takes away a leg he finally realizes will never grow back again.

In some miraculous way, a child is expected to cope with these disasters because, so he is told, they are for his own good. But unlike adults, a small child cannot intellectualize or interpret them in spiritual or philosophical terms. Yet children are expected to behave stoically so as not to upset the staff or their parents. The mother says to her child after a painful procedure during which the child was restrained by two adults, "Thank the doctor, dear." And the child mumbles thanks to the doctor who does the best he can to pull his own shattered nerves together. One must ask, however, why haven't these doctors called on their scientific brethren in pharmacology and psychology to develop medicines and methods that would ameliorate the trauma of these devastating procedures?

Even the process by which anticancer drugs are fed into the veins is a distressing business. The veins of children, small to begin with, weakened by the disease, are apt to collapse, one reason that children with leukemia are often covered with black and blue marks from weak blood vessels breaking beneath the skin. After a while, the only veins that can be used for injecting anticancer drugs may be in the scalp. To the child with leukemia, humiliated by his hairlessness, there then is the added punishment of a needle inserted in his scalp and science-fiction tubes extending from it. No verbal protests come from children subjected to this indignity, this Martian-like freakish image. But they express their suppressed rage in drawings, caricatures of themselves. Sometimes they get back at the grown-ups responsible for this outrage by drawing big people with shaved heads and needles stuck in *their* scalps and long loops of tubes scrawling all over the paper.

In hospitals where procedures take precedence over people, it is too easy to disregard the sensitivities of patients, especially children who are unlikely to complain to hospital administrators. Their helplessness and low status deprive them even of simple courtesies. A little girl, only 3 years old, sobbed uncontrollably in the arms of Susan Castelluccio because, as the child explained between sobs, "They cut the sleeve of my pink shirt. They didn't take it off to put the needle in. They cut it right here." The child showed the blood-stained sleeve that had been thoughtlessly cut to insert the needle for a blood transfusion. "I'll fix it," said Miss Castelluccio. And she took the child's pink shirt home, sewed the sleeve together, and washed the shirt in a bowl with a pink shirt of her own.

The next day, wearing her own pink shirt, she put the mended one on the little girl and told her she had washed it with her own, and that now they were both wearing their clean pink shirts. "Oh, Susan," the child exclaimed ecstatically, hugging the young therapist, "You fixed it. And you washed it with yours!"

Pain and unhappiness had been banished not only by the mended sleeve, but by that 3-year-old child's appreciation of the exquisite courtesy an adult had displayed toward her, the lovely intimacy of the two pink shirts together in the wash bowl. That child had endured without protest loneliness and misery, the violence of medicines, confinement to a hospital bed, but she had been broken down by the heedlessness of grown-ups to whom a little pink sleeve was of no importance.

The stoicism of many children is not grounded in

strong character, but in terror. They don't cry or wince, are cooperative with doctors and nurses because they are afraid that if they don't conceal their suffering, even more pain might be inflicted on them in new kinds of treatment. When directly questioned by parents or doctors, a child may feel threatened and refuse to give any information. But, when confronted by one of his art productions and the easy, apparently aimless questions of an art therapist, the child will explain what is happening inside him. "It is easier," say Susan Castelluccio, "to talk about the sad monster in a drawing or the broken machine than to talk about one's sadness or the broken machine that is one's own body. They can draw a figure with a leg or arm missing, but they can't talk about their own lost limb. Even at a very early age, children are sensitive about disfigurement. While they're in the hospital, there is a common understanding among them, unspoken sympathy for other children worse off. But outside the hospital, when they return to school, go to play areas, or to the movies, or on outings, they discover the terrible stigma of disfigurement, tumors that have distorted a face, a missing arm or leg, and the hairless head. Yet, despite their amputations and disfigurements, these children display a life force that is heart gripping."

A needle jabbed into your fingertip during your annual checkup is not especially traumatic, though you may wince and look away as the needle goes into the skin for the blood sample. But if your fingertips were pricked every day, day after day, week after week, you would most likely dread the procedure.

"Taking blood samples from children with leukemia was as traumatic for me as for them," Vivian Dickson, a former medical technologist, told me. "When I went into the room with my tray of needles and syringes, the child would visibly tense, then hold up the little hands, spreading the fingers like spokes to show me on each finger an arch of tiny red marks. I always tried to find a spot that had no sign of a puncture mark. Talking to the child as I took the sample helped a little. They usually grimaced and sometimes averted their faces as I stuck the lancet in the fingertip, then they'd watch fascinated as the blood rushed into the tiny tube. As I dabbed their fingers afterwards with antiseptic, I'd say, 'Now, that really didn't hurt that much, did it?' and they'd usually nod their heads, agreeing with me. But I knew, of course, that it wasn't merely a matter of pricking a finger and drawing a blood sample three or four times a week. The procedure had dreaded implications for those children. Even those who are quite young are very sophisticated about their disease. They know that if the sample shows that the platelet count is low, they will have to undergo the much more painful procedure of bone marrow aspiration. So, taking the blood sample is part of a threatening sequence and the children always reflect their anxiety."

The anxiety and pain of finger sticking shows up in the children's drawings. As common among their drawings as the flaming, crashing plane following "Bone Day" is the figure of a hairless child with enormous disproportionate hands, thick splayed fingers, blood red. Long spears point diagonally at the fingers, sometimes merely menacing, sometimes piercing a finger.

Miss Castelluccio sits with a child and admires his drawing. The child is pleased. They talk about the picture. Yes, he is the little figure and that spear is the needle jabbed into one of the huge red fingers. Yes, the needle hurts every time. It gets worse. All his fingers hurt all the time. He doesn't have enough skin left for the next hole that will have to be punctured. He knows no one wants to hurt him, but they do. Every few days they have to take the blood and look at it through a glass to see if the medicine is killing the bad cells. But painful as the finger jab is, he'd rather have that than the bone jab.

Dr. Lucius Sinks says that there are ways of helping children with cancer pain to cope with it. "Telling them about the mechanics of treatment is one way. It helps especially youngsters in their early teens. At that age, the imagination goes wild. The more children understand, the better they can cope. Some older pediatricians believe in keeping back information from children. They think children should not be told the facts about their disease, that they should be protected from that knowledge. But in the last 10 or 15 years, when treatment was being developed that held out some hope for control of the disease, it has been the policy of younger doctors to be open with the children and with their parents. There are still some physicians who can't cope with the helplessness of the situation and feel so uncomfortable themselves that they can't talk about it with children or parents."

At Children's Hospital National Medical Center in Washington, D.C., a 13-year-old girl, talking with Sandra Butcher, social worker at the hospital, told her how she wished the leukemia blood testing procedures could be carried out. It would be much better, the child said, if her parents told her ahead of time that there would be a spinal tap or bone marrow test. But coming into the hospital on a routine visit and then suddenly being told there would be a spinal tap or bone marrow test didn't give her enough time to "build up" to accepting the pain. Children should know beforehand what is going to take place so they can condition themselves. Even waiting for the finger stick of the needle for drawing blood can be scary.

When Mrs. Butcher asked her, "What do you think the doctor should do?" the child replied, "I think he should talk about the procedure, explain it while he's doing it because that helps keep your mind off the pain. He should tell everything he's doing as he goes along, everything, even about the cold rag. [A cloth soaked in alcohol to sterilize the skin where the needle will be inserted.]

"And I wish all the painful procedures could be done in quick succession, all the same day. But first they draw the blood from your finger, then they test the blood to find out what the cell count is and then you get treatment. It seems to take hours for that and you wait, not knowing for sure what's going to happen. Then, if there's a problem about the cells, you have to have more tests. Sometimes I feel almost like a doctor, telling myself about the pain and how long the procedures take. It takes about ten minutes to get out the bone marrow from the time the needle goes into the bone and it's a bad experience every time. In four years, there were only two I didn't feel. When I said to the nurse how easy one of them was, she said, 'They won't always be that easy.' I know she meant well, that she didn't want me to expect all the tests to be easy, but I couldn't help worrying about the next ones."

Enshrined in this little girl's heart is the technologist who usually drew the blood sample from her finger. "She sort of takes the pain for you, saying 'Ouch!' and twisting up her face and doing all the things you feel like doing when it hurts. And she looks so funny, you can't help laughing and when you're laughing you're not feeling the pain and then it's all over."

In an interview, Mrs. Butcher said to me, "There are two faces of pediatric pain. There's the child's pain and there's the pain of the parents who see their children suffering and are helpless to do anything about it. Parents of children who have leukemia have to find their own way of coping with it. Some of them don't tell the children what their disease is, but the children usually find out. One father told his son that the disease was anemia. But, of course, the boy found out shortly after he came into the hospital. Most children discover that the more they know about what's happening and how they're likely to react, the better they handle their reactions. They find out that what they feel is pretty much the way the other children feel, too. Some children understand instinctively that part of the reason their parents don't tell them the truth about their disease is that the parents have a desperate need to deceive themselves. Even after children discover the truth, they often keep the secret to spare their parents. This double deception causes great confusion in the relationship until the truth finally comes out into the open."

But Mrs. Butcher believes that there is something to be said for not knowing too much too soon. "It can cause excessive apprehension on both sides. Sometimes the deception, the ruses practiced to deceive each other, allow the initial shock and trauma to be attenuated somewhat so that when everyone faces the truth together, there has been a period of preparation for it."

Cultural patterns, followed and accepted for generations in a different country and setting, can run headlong into disaster when a grave illness develops in a child. Mrs. Butcher told of a situation that occurred in a family that came to the United States from a country where traditionally the raising of children is the total responsibility of the mother until the boys become adolescents. Then the father takes over, guiding and instructing his sons. The 11-year-old boy in this family developed a tumor on the brainstem. He was operated on, most of the tumor was removed, and, after a painful convalescence, was taken home. But within months, he felt pain in his head. More tumor. The boy begged his father not to send him back to the hospital for more surgery, but the father was determined that his son be cured. If surgery was the only way, the boy must undergo it. The major tumor mass was removed, but, again, after some months there was regrowth. Evident to everyone, including the boy, was that the malignancy could not be controlled. But the father, obsessed by grief and disappointment, could not accept the fact. Nor could he listen to his son, pleading to remain at home, begging his father not to send him back to the hospital again. It was only after Mrs. Butcher talked with the father and urged him to listen to his son that the father finally heard not merely the doomed boy's words, but beneath them, the boy's understanding of his condition.

The father, surmounting his desperate desire to have his son made whole and healthy, accepted the fact that the boy would not grow into manhood, would never go through the traditional rearing years, the close period of father-son guidance. With only weeks, possibly months left for sharing, the father took his son home from the hospital for the last time. He bought a walkie-talkie set and during the day, while working on his construction job, he talked with his son at home, even teaching him the language of the old country. No longer fearful of more surgery and pain and anxiety over being separated from the comforting presence of his mother and brothers and sisters, the boy turned to his father in a relationship quite different from the traditional one in the old country, but deeper, closer, and more loving.

Whether to leave a child in the hospital or take him or her home is one of the anguishing dilemmas parents face. What the very young child wants even more than to get well—for that can be a vague concept to a 4-year-old—is to go home. Face to face with a medical team committed to using every possible means of treatment, parents can be overwhelmed by the burden of choice. It is in these situations, when treatment must be weighed against the quality of the child's life during its final stages, that social workers, by listening carefully to the patient, the family, the nurses, and the doctors help families choose a solution best suited to their particular situation. Sometimes, the decision is to take the child home where he or she is free of the discomforts of the aggressive treatment and the strictures of hospital routine. Even though parents make this decision rationally and with guidance, some parents are fearful of what relatives and others might say about their decision. They want to be absolutely sure that what they are doing is not "odd" or in any way an abnormal thing to do.

They fear, and not unreasonably, the criticisms of relatives and perhaps neighbors. Such fears are not to be lightly brushed aside by anyone on the medical team, for they often symbolize feelings of guilt, irrational as they may be, that torment parents of children who have cancer. When obviously continuing treatment cannot help the child, a nurse or social worker trusted by the parents gives the reassurance they need, helping them to shift their concern over the opinions of outsiders to the comfort of their dying child.

On the face of it, taking a dying child home to spend his or her final days in an atmosphere of consoling attention would seem the final gesture of love. But resistance sometimes arises from unexpected sources. It is normal for brothers and sisters to resent secretly a cossetted child, but a jealous grandmother? Here one encounters the fallacy of the stereotypes: Grandmothers are always loving and indulgent to their grandchildren. Not always, it seems, as a young couple discovered when they took their 3-year-old son home from the hospital after doctors said his cancer was incurable and that he would live only a few weeks. A few days after the child arrived home, the grandmother, a partial invalid who lived with the family, developed heart flutters. Distraught, the parents went back to the hospital to talk the problem over with Mrs. Butcher, who knew the family, and she suggested that a little more attention to grandmother might cure the heart flutters. And so it turned out. Once the grandmother was reassured that her own care was not being disregarded and that family concern could be divided between her and her dying grandson, her health improved and the flutters stopped.

A study of the benefits and limitations of taking dying children home from the hospital was carried out under the auspices of the University of Minnesota School of Nursing. According to Dr. Ida Martinson, director of the study, they were looking for answers to such questions as: What are the most immediate problems for the child and other family members during home care? What does the child see as the benefits and limitations of home care? What values or disadvantages do the rest of the family see in home care? How do home-care costs compare with hospital care?

When this book was being written, the study was at its halfway mark. Dr. Martinson reported at the American Cancer Society's Nineteenth Science Writers' Seminar that all the children, except one, in the study suffered cancer-related pain. "According to our findings thus far," Dr. Martinson said, "it seems that pain can be as well controlled at home as in the hospital. This may indicate that the hospital is perhaps not essential for providing the comfort care needed by a dying child. If so, this fact must be recognized by all of the four major participants—the physician, the nurse, the parents, and the child. The physician may need to allow some flexibility in pain management for the nurse and family. The nurse must be knowledgeable regarding pain control, for she appears to be a major factor in the maintenance of pain control in the home. The parents must realize that pain can be as well controlled at home or they will unnecessarily take the child to the hospital for pain control."

One child who went back to the hospital for pain medication was given three injections of morphine sulfate, which could have been administered at home. To allay his apprehension, the child should be told that pain can be controlled at home. Pain control is particularly important at night not only for the child, but to ensure some uninterrupted sleep for the family. Pain medication which is effective for a six- to eight-hour period is therefore preferred.

"Other than this project," Dr. Martinson said, "there appears to be no organized effort to study the feasibility and desirability of home care for the dying child, although attempts are being made to provide a home-like atmosphere in the hospital. Another current approach deals with the concept of the hospice, which is currently limited to adult patients."

As this study showed, besides the emotional benefits to the child and the family, there are striking economic advantages to home care of the dying child. "In a chart audit done in January 1977, of 12 children with cancer who died in the hospital, total actual last-hospitalization costs averaged $12,000 per child," said Dr. Martinson. "By contrast, the average cost for the 11 children who died at home was less than $700."

Children, like adults, develop their own pain games. Who knows the secret reason a little boy in obvious pain denies it, shaking his head, saying over and over again, "No pain, no pain." Often this kind of denial is a screen a child throws up when he is soon to go home from the hospital and doesn't want anything to interfere with that departure. So, to be safe, though hurting, he says, "I don't hurt, honest."

Some children become adept at using pain to manipulate others. Occasionally it's a poignant attempt to bring together parents who have separated, the child hoping his suffering will heal their wounds. Or a fractious, angry, frustrated child may tyrannize parents and hospital staff with complaints about pain, which may or may not be present. Behavioral scientists have learned much about adults who use pain for personal advantage, but there haven't been studies of how this type of behavior gets started very early in children. The pain behavior of children, forerunner of so many behavioral problems that later turn up in pain clinics, has yet to be explored.

The child picks up from parents ways of reacting to pain—stoically, cravenly, plaintively. Besides the manner in which reactions to pain are expressed, there are the parents' attitudes toward pain, a form of atonement for real or imagined sins, or a terrible injustice, or as a way of identifying with the sufferings of Christ, or a form of prepayment for a direct passage to heaven. And for a few, pain is treated as a nuisance to be ignored because there are important things to be done.

Whatever the concepts of his parents—and two parents may have conflicting concepts—the child incorporates something of those attitudes in his own concepts. He will have a smattering of guilt, for he has very early experienced the heady feeling of power in disobedience and its aftermath, guilt. Very young children who suffer from prolonged illness or serious injuries consider it punishment, not necessarily for anything specific, but for having been "bad" at one time or another.

Little children have no inhibitions about expressing their pain—they yell and scream. But in "middle childhood," that limbo between 8 and 12, children's ways of coping with pain reveal their social training. Nancy V. Schultz, pediatric nurse, found in her study[1] of middle-class preteenage boys and girls, black and white, that beneath their control of strong feelings, not far below the surface, was their need for support and reassurance. Eight of the 74 children she studied admitted that they responded to pain by crying. Twenty-one boys labeled themselves "brave," but only 4 girls so described themselves. All the girls admitted to being nervous and afraid in painful situations and 28 boys frankly confessed to fear and anxiety. Some of the boys and girls said that though they felt like crying when in pain, they held it back.

Mrs. Schultz comments that nurses and society expect boys to be brave and that it is acceptable for boys to feel like crying, provided they don't. Boys in middle childhood are expected to be "strong, assertive, and courageous." Later on they are expected to suppress fear and, under stress, to control their emotions. Girls are allowed, even encouraged to show fear, hurt feelings, and general emotional upsets.

In middle childhood, boys and girls are taking their first steps toward independence. Those who become afflicted with chronic pain from cancer or injuries suffer an added dimension in the conflict between wanting to cry from the almost unbearable pain and the fear of slipping back into infantile dependence. As a result, says Mrs. Schultz, children of this age may go to great lengths to conceal their suffering, physical and emotional. Stoicism should not be interpreted by the medical team as nonsuffering, as it often is "sometimes at great emotional cost to the child."

When asked about the meaning of pain, the children in Mrs. Schultz's study related it to death. In a hospital, this fear can grow irrationally. What these young patients may be telling the medical team may be something quite different from what the team members think they are hearing. Even in middle childhood, beset as it is with anxieties, frustrations, and conflict, independence is a dominant need and pain deprives those children of control. When pain is lessened, independence is strengthened. "Pain," says Mrs. Schultz, "isn't just a broken leg, or an injection; it is also growing, changing, being scolded, failing in school, and not having visitors."

To what extent infants experience pain is an open question. Doctors who deliver babies think the baby's howl when smacked on the bottom is a pain response. Dr. Alfred L. Florman, pediatrician at New York University Medical Center, says that anyone who has seen the new born baby's response to a slap on the soles of his feet or on his buttocks cannot doubt that the newborn experiences pain. At this early age when sensitivity is not so acute as it is later, only a strong stimulus elicits a response. For example, a newborn's clavicle may be fractured during labor, but unlike the older child with a similar injury, the baby rarely cries because of the fracture, which may be overlooked unless the pediatrician specifically looks for it during his examination.

Janet Steiger, Wisconsin mother, drawing on her own child-rearing experience, says that before a child learns to speak, he expresses pain through sounds and body language. "Crying, the classic symptom of discomfort, can signal anything from wet diapers to severe illness. Parents usually develop a certain sensitivity to the differences in the child's cries. If feeding, burping, rocking, or distracting toys stop the crying, parents assume they have taken care of the cause. But if a child continues to cry, then parents check for fever, teething, rash, pallor, or lethargy, all possible indicators of pain-producing problems.

"The absence of crying may in some cases be an indicator of serious trouble. The baby who simply whimpers, or is silently unresponsive may be suffering more severe pain than the shrieker. Wise mothers say: They really worry me when they're too quiet.

"If a child does not cry, but keeps pulling at his ear lobe, or rubs it continuously, it may be a signal of an ear infection. A baby who thrashes about may be experiencing the acute pain of colic. Any change in motion patterns should alert a mother to possible trouble that a child cannot express in words. A growing baby's behavior patterns do change, of course, but a sudden reversal of usual behavior or persistent motion with signs of distress should be watched as a possible pain-related problem."

In industrial countries, burns are the most common type of injuries in children. Their world is filled with all manner of appliances—stoves, sometimes poorly insulated, with enticing circles of blue flames or glowing, orange coils. There are electric coffeepots, heaters, grills, hot plates, warmers, handles to be grasped and pots of boiling liquid tipped over, and the magic of matches. In living rooms, unguarded open fires, in cellars heaters that explode. And arsonists. And drunk, deranged adults who torture children with lighted cigarettes and boiling water.

Against a background film of a flaming house, a television newsman says, "Property damage is estimated at $20,000. One child survived and is hospitalized with second-degree burns covering 60 percent of his body." Consider for a moment what that means: 60 percent of the body's surface. Multiply by 60 the damage to your fingertip if you held it for one minute in the flame of a stove gas burner. Relate that to the child with 60 percent of the body burned, flesh and nerves raw. What areas of the child were burned? Is the face recognizable or is it like a small ball of melted wax? Will the child be able to use his hands again or are ligaments permanently damaged? Were the boy's genitals destroyed? Will he be blind?

First-degree burns in which the outer layer of the skin gets red and may blister are, as most of us know, extremely sensitive and may hurt for days. Second-degree burns, in which nerves are damaged, are excruciatingly painful, require expert care to prevent infection, and are slow to heal. In the most serious types of burns, third degree, skin and nerves are destroyed and must be covered by skin grafts. The more extensive the body area burned, the more likely the burn is to be fatal. There is a massive loss of fluids, sometimes lung damage, stomach ulcers, malfunctioning of most of the body organs. The rate at which the body converts food into energy speeds up like a fire in a strong draft. Only by greatly increasing his food intake can a burned person compensate for this accelerated metabolism. Scientists only recently are finding out why burns disrupt bodily functions and how to counteract them.

Each year 29 percent of children under 15 who have

been burned on 30 percent or more of their body surface die. Deep burns, hideous as their scars are, especially those that disfigure the face and defy even the great skills of caring, dedicated plastic surgeons, do more than visible damage. They destroy muscles and ligaments. When only partial restoration is possible, the result may be clawlike hands, arms that cannot be raised above the shoulder, legs and feet that move only by shuffling, or an empty eye socket.

Only the intractable pain of terminal cancer, which also involves damage to the nerves, is considered as frightful as the pain of serious burns. But the pain of the burn itself is more than matched by the treatment for it. Patients who recoil from even a feather touch are scrubbed with brushes to remove dead skin and undergo the agony of tubbing where roiling water stimulates the burned area. Splints with wires are put on arms and legs to stretch retracted muscles to prevent joints from stiffening or the limb from atrophying. Skin grafts, usually transferring skin from one part of the body of the burned person, cause pain in the area from which the skin is removed; the patient, then, suffers from two sources of pain—the burn itself and the graft.

"The situation in which a burn occurs has a lot to do with how a child reacts to pain," Judith Kruter, R.N., former coordinator of the burn unit at the Children's Hospital Medical Center in Washington, D.C., said in an interview. "Children who, though badly burned, survive a fire, but lose one or both parents suffer far more intensely from pain than burned children whose parents survive the fire.

"The children who have an extraordinary tolerance for pain are the ones who have been deliberately tortured, immersed in boiling water, or put on heated electric hot plates, or burned in other ways, and who have been repeatedly abused. They've learned that screaming from pain often meant that beating and battering and burning would be repeated in retaliation for their cries of pain and distress. In our burn unit, these children endure the pain of the burn itself stoically and scarcely whimper during treatment which can be excruciating. About 15 to 20 percent of the children in this burn unit have been deliberately burned by adults."

Mrs. Kruter said that burned adults can be motivated to endure terrible pain in therapy because they know how important it is to restore movement in arms and legs and feet. "But children, especially very small children, cannot project into the future and see the permanent handicaps they could have if the use of their limbs isn't restored. We encourage the children to exercise the muscles of their arms and hands by feeding themselves though that may be very difficult and painful to do. We have special games and toys that require movement of the muscles that have been injured by the burns. From the moment a child is brought into the burn unit, a therapist is called in to evaluate the damage to the child's joints and muscles and to plan an exercise program."

Nurses in the burn unit explain to the children who are old enough to understand why they must take the painful whirlpool baths, what the bubbles do to help them get better, and the reason for the splints. But the children's pain and anxiety are sometimes so intense that they cannot hear with their minds these explanations of the value of the treatments. Nor can some cooperate in their treatment by submitting without resistance to changes of dressings and removal of dead tissue.

If burned children either deliberately or accidentally

set the fire, or in any way contributed to the disaster that injured them, they are apt to feel a strong sense of guilt and to associate the pain with deserved punishment. Even if a child is burned in a car accident or in an explosion, or in any other situation for which he had no responsibility, he may nevertheless consider the burn and pain punishment for some imagined crime or sin.

Nurses encourage children to cry during the agonizing debridement treatment when dead, burned skin is cut away or scrubbed off or during the painful tubbings. "It's difficult for the nurses to be the ones who must cause so much suffering in the course of the treatment," said Mrs. Kruter. "In order not to be associated with only the painful aspects of the hospital experiences, our nurses read to the children, play games with them, and feed them when necessary. And the children's rooms are sanctuaries from inflicted pain. In them no painful procedures are carried out. We want the children to associate their rooms with pleasant things, games and good things to eat, and stories to listen to."

Because of the fast rate at which a severely burned body metabolizes food, it's essential that patients eat a lot of food to replace the vital losses. Burned children who are beyond the infant stage understand this. "But," Mrs. Kruter said, "the child's need to exert some control or to punish those whose intentions are the best, but whose treatment causes such anguish sometimes warps his behavior. To control others, or punish them, or merely to rebel, children, though well aware of how important food is to their recovery, become adept at vomiting their meals. It's not unusual for a nurse to spend a long time coaxing a child to eat all the food on the tray, getting him to respond to her solicitous attention, especially a nurse who is anxious to eradicate from the child's mind the horror of a debridement, and, after what she believes was a successful feeding session, to start to leave the room and, when she gets as far as the foot of the bed, the child vomits the meal all over it. Many children can do that at will and fearlessly, for they know nothing worse can be done to them than the punishment they take every day in being treated."

Some children who cannot cooperate in their treatment may be given Valium or other tranquilizers to reduce anxiety and relax their muscles. But pain control for children, Mrs. Kruter feels, is one of the great lacks in medicine.

Physicians generally say quite confidently that pain in children can be controlled adequately by adapting analgesics designed for adults. But as one pediatric nurse expressed it: "If you relate the dose to the age and size of the child, you may have to cut an aspirin into 12 pieces and one-twelfth of an aspirin isn't likely to help a child who is in agony from an arthritic flare-up, or a child with bone tumor, or one whose burned skin has to be scraped away. As for using morphine or Demerol for pain control in a very little child, the amount you can use safely is so small that it scarcely wets the needle. But the general attitude toward relieving pain in children is that when something seems to work why bother to improve it. Nobody asks how well it works or why aren't there analgesics specifically for the severe, prolonged pain children suffer today because the treatment enables them to survive what would have killed them a few years ago."

Some members of the health-care team explain the lack of interest in the suffering of children in this way: A child is easier to ignore than an adult. A child cannot take his complaint to the head nurse or to the hospital administrator. A child does not write indignant letters to the editor of the local newspaper revealing the callous treatment he received in the local hospital. Nor does a child bring consumer action against the hospital for causing his undue suffering. Though children write millions of letters to their congressmen asking for information, they do not write to them about the indifference of the medical profession to the almost insupportable pain some children needlessly endure.

By screams, spasms of pain, and writhings, the helpless, very small child articulates his agony, usually to no avail. A young physician, taking a few months of pediatric training in a hospital, was changing the dressing of a horribly burned little girl who screamed in agony. One of the three attending nurses, unnerved by the child's cries, suggested to the young doctor that perhaps the child should be given something to calm her. His reply: "There are three of you to hold her."

The isolation of burned children is another element in their suffering. The dangers of infection in the burned area are so serious that only parents are allowed to visit. Occasionally, extraordinary circumstances justify breaking this hospital rule, as in the instance of two brothers who were the only survivors when their house was destroyed by fire. The two boys, both in grave condition, were taken to different hospitals, one to the Children's Hospital National Medical Center. He had burns over 70 percent of his body and was not expected to live. He grieved constantly for his dead parents and his absent brother. When the brother who had been less seriously burned was released from the hospital, he was taken to the bedside of his brother who seemed likely to die. The reunion of the two little boys revived the still hospitalized child's will to survive. He recovered.

Burn wards are not quiet places. Sudden screams bring nurses running. A fitfully sleeping child has torn off the bandages and wakens fully to the agonizing pain from exposed wounds. Other children waken. One sobs uncontrollably. Piercing cries of fear and anxiety. Nurses hush and comfort, mostly with words, for severely and extensively burned children cannot be cradled in consoling arms.

Dr. Alia Y. Antoon, assistant pediatrician at the Shriners Burns Institute in Boston, said in an interview that the "noise level" (screaming, crying, yelling) in most hospital burn units is high. "Since the Institute opened a few years ago and we have this place for burned children only, the noise level has been significantly lower. Before the Burn Institute was opened, burned children were admitted on the general pediatric floor of the Massachusetts General Hospital. The reduction in noise level is due to the training and education of the staff and the success in treatment techniques which bring hope into the care of some of the most seriously burned children. When the unit was part of a general hospital, nurses were treating patients who had other types of problems and were not specializing in pain control. Here at the Institute, there is no scrubbing or tubbing, two extremely painful procedures that are not only terribly distressing to the children, but to the nurses who go through the ordeal with them. Older children are especially anxious about the effects of burns on their appearance and on their ability to function."

From her own experience with burned children, Dr. Antoon sees a need for studies of different analgesics, comparing certain mild ones like aspirin with sedatives like chloral hydrate, a sleep-inducing drug, and antihistamines to find out how safe and effective these different medications are. She also advocates studies on ways of improving the interaction between staff and the children. The physical environment and the psychological ambience are especially important in the care of burned children.

"Interactions between staff and the children greatly influence recovery. We know from our experience here that nurses who are relaxed and confident get better cooperation from the children. Trained volunteers, too, play an important role as part of the team. They read to the children, talk with them, and divert them with games. Another influence on recovery is how well physicians and nurses explain to children what is happening, why certain painful procedures are necessary. Explaining such things to very small children requires special skills in communication, but it's surprising how well most children cooperate when they understand. If we had a better understanding of the techniques of staff-patient interactions, we could perhaps improve staff training. The turnover rate of the well trained staff caring for burned children in an environment especially designed for children with burns is lower than in the general hospital."

The Burns Institute in Boston is one of three established by the Shriners of North America, the other two in Cincinnati and Galveston. In all three, care of burned children is tied in with research on the many aspects of burns. Specially selected and trained staffs give the finest medical care to children who come from immediate areas, from other parts of the United States, and some from foreign countries. In the treatment program, the "whole child" is considered, his or her future, the family, the psychological and emotional impact of serious burns, and the restoration, as much as possible, of activity to damaged hands, arms, legs and feet. The Institute admits burned infants and children 15 years or younger regardless of the extent of the burn or the family's income. The Institute's treatment program includes medical care, surgery, and rehabilitation.

Medical teams in each of the Shriners burns institutes include surgeons with special skills in plastic and orthopedic surgery, pediatricians, nurses, anesthesiologists, psychiatrists, psychologists, social workers, bio-chemists, microbiologists, physical and recreational therapists, school teachers, and trained volunteers. At the Boston Institute, about 100 acutely burned children are admitted each year and treatment is given annually to about 400, many of them children who return for additional plastic surgery and therapy. Some children continue their treatment into adulthood.

Surgical techniques developed at the Boston Institute make possible skin grafts over the burned areas as early as the third day after the burn, without waiting for the burned tissue to slough or be scrubbed off. This early grafting speeds recovery, reduces pain in the burn itself, and spares the child some of the distressing treatment procedures.

Research at the Institute centers on studies of crippling contractures caused by damaged muscles, wound healing, regeneration of nerves and tissue, metabolism, immunology, the graft rejection phenomena, anesthetics, as well as the circulatory and respiratory problems common to burned people. Information from the studies is applied in treatment, helping reduce trauma and pain. "The application of successful techniques makes taking care of the children more rewarding to the nurses," said Dr. Antoon. "And the supportive services of social workers and volunteers reduce suffering and subsequent impairment."

Despite heroic efforts of plastic surgeons at the Shriners Burns Institute to restore a severely burned face, in some instances totally reconstructing it, the new face rarely resembles the original one. It is beyond the powers of any unscarred person to imagine the anguish a child, especially a young teenager, suffers because of his mutilated face. In his book, *Emotional Care of the Facially Burned and Disfigured,* Dr. Norman R. Bernstein, psychiatrist at the Shriners Burns Institute in Boston, tells the story of a teenage boy who, after a long, harrowing hospital stay, during which numerous plastic surgery operations had been performed to restore his severely burned face, returned home to become a recluse, only venturing out in darkness. His mother finally persuaded him to accompany her on a visit to one of her friends, who had been prepared for the boy's terrible disfigurement. During the visit, the teenage daughter of the hostess came unexpectedly into the room. Horrified, she stared at the boy's face, and, convinced he was playing a joke, wearing a mask to frighten her, went to him to pull it off, then suddenly realized it was the boy's real face.

New staff members, especially nurses, assailed by screams for mercy during dressing changes, wrenched by the helplessness of the children and their fear of dying, go through a period of depression themselves in their first months on duty. Dr. Bernstein, as he recounts in his book, suggested hypnosis for improving the children's cooperativeness, pain tolerance, and appetite, which, in turn, would benefit the nurses in their work. His predictions were fulfilled: The children responded to this form of therapy, formerly discouraged nurses approached their work with hope and enthusiasm, and patient and staff morale improved markedly.

Burned children have a great need to be touched, Dr. Bernstein writes, but "bandages, isolation units, masks, charred and desensitized skin all interfere with bodily communication and physical contact.... Hypnotic induction with them is particularly easy when there is physical contact because they are so eager for it. Their physical discomfort makes them desperate to escape into the trance state. Once members of the staff begin to see that they can communicate with children in physical ways, they do so and ask less for hypnosis, which is then seen as a competitor for intimacy. The degree of illness definitely makes a difference; all severely burned individuals have a major threat to their lives and undergo exquisite agony, repeated surgery, and many frightening procedures. The multiple traumatic experiences and the massive assaults following 50 to 60 percent burns require forceful coping mechanisms ... perhaps it is for this reason that we have never seen burned adults or children during [hypnotic] induction nor seen staff or patients regard hypnosis as a hazard. Parents have never interfered, if only because the permission required is so much less threatening than that needed for amputations or skin grafting (often with the parents as donors), and hypnosis also lightens the burden of emotional support. 'We'll agree to *anything* that will help,' parents often declare."[2]

Even after the novelty of hypnosis wears off, Dr. Bernstein finds that it continues to be useful, mostly for patients in physical therapy who are frightened or uncooperative. And it helps some children express feelings of guilt and grief, especially those who have been in any way responsible for a fire in which other members of the family were injured or killed.

It is strange that, among the untold millions the federal government and private agencies spend on the care of mentally retarded and deformed children, practically nothing is spent to relieve the pain and anguish of burned and injured children. Physicians concentrate on a disease, or broken bones, or a burn itself. Pediatricians give papers at annual meetings on anomalies, deformities, ambiguities, new surgical techniques, and much about organs and systems. At the last three meetings of the American Academy of Pediatrics, there was not one paper among hundreds on controlling pain in children. Physicians and nurses can speak of "noise levels" as if the sounds emanated from stereo sets, tapes or recordings, not from desperate, lonely, anxious little human beings. The professionals on the medical team who voice their concern in journals are nurses.

In her article, "Pain Relief for the Child,"[3] Margo McCaffery, R.N., says that regarding pain in general, the nurse is primarily accountable for two aspects: reporting pain that might have significance in the child's illness, and controlling "the child's expression of pain." That phrase means keeping the child quiet, something Mrs. McCaffery says can be done "without providing pain relief." Nurses can ignore crying and screaming, can punish with disapproving looks, or admonish a child to be brave, behavioral control techniques that sometimes work even with very small children. "Behavior control without pain relief," says Mrs. McCaffery, "can make the pain experience a truly horrifying one for the child.

"No one on the health team is accountable for providing pain relief. However, the nurse spends more time with the child in pain than does any other member of the health team. For this reason, among others, it seems that the nurse should examine carefully his/her role in pain relief."

Complicating the pain control situation is the fact that physicians and nurses use manifestations of acute pain as the basis for judging all pain. Sudden, intense pain may produce observable changes in respiration, sweating, pulse rate, or pallor. The suffering person may weep or scream, fight off attendants attempting to staunch blood or bandage him. "When pain persists for hours or days, or sometimes for even a few minutes," says Mrs. McCaffery, "a process of adaptation occurs. Physiological parameters return to near normal. Changes in response to sudden and severe pain, such as rapid pulse, cannot be sustained without harm to the body."

Besides making this physiological adaptation, children may adapt to continuing pain by controlling their expressions of it to measure up to "expectations of parents or nurses, or because of personal values in the case of the older child." If a child has not been raised in the stoical tradition, he quickly learns that it is expected of him in the hospital. Even a child suffering severely, when too tired to cry or rock or complain, will drop into an exhausted sleep, misleading those about him into thinking that his pain could not have been too bad.

"It is commonly said that children require less frequent administration of analgesics and for shorter periods of time than adults do with comparable pathology," Mrs. McCaffery says. "This conclusion may be reached erroneously because the child is much less able than the adult to communicate his pain in a manner we recognize."

Radical in medical practice, but very much in tune with the times, is Mrs. McCaffery's suggestions that nurses "express a desire to collaborate with the child and the parents in planning pain relief. The child as young as two years old may be able to identify something that would help him cope with a painful event, such as holding mommy's hand or clinging to a stuffed animal. Parents usually have handled numerous brief episodes of pain with their child. They possess a wealth of information that can be used to individualize the plan for pain relief."

Not all the pain problems of children are confined to the hospital setting. A possible reason that dentists have a higher suicide rate than other health professionals may be the hell they go through with terrified children. I still remember the horror chamber that was our dentist's office, the big brown leather chair, menacing instruments lined up in full view behind the glass door of his cabinet, and the gas mask pressed over my face. And the time the gas didn't last long enough and in his haste to finish, the dentist losing his grip on the tooth, and the sensation as it slipped down my throat.

The new generation of dentists caters to children, assuaging their apprehension through bright colors, cheerful, amusing prints on the walls, games to play while the children await their turn, and in some offices soothing music. Gone are the somber, rigid chairs that evoked images of prison electrocutions, and the rows of gruesome instruments exposed behind glass cabinet doors. In their place are pastel-colored versions of the chaise longue and cabinets of drawers you can't see through.

And young dentists are more sophisticated in dealing with scared children. Dr. Joseph Penn, a Bethesda, Maryland, dentist, uses the imaginations of his children patients as an anesthetic. Before starting work on their teeth, he tells them to watch their favorite television program, to see it in their mind's eye, and when the commercial comes on to raise one arm. Sometimes, intent on his work, he is puzzled when a child slowly raises his or her arm. Ah, yes, the commercial.

As a substitute for anesthetics, dentists used to stuff a towel into a youngster's mouth until he calmed down.

Others have chased hysterical children around the office and when they caught them, jabbed an injection of anesthetic into their bottoms. For extracting teeth from children, some dentists used—and some still do—a general anesthetic, a risky procedure for any child. Even more dangerous, says a research scientist in dental anesthesiology, "is the practice of augmenting a light general anesthetic with an injection of a local anesthetic containing epinephrine into an angry, terrified child whose system is pouring out hormones that may interact with the drug combination with potentially fatal results." This same scientist says that urgently needed "is research in the entire pain and anxiety control system in dentistry and along with that an adequate pain control and training program in dental schools."

Aside from humanitarian reasons for controlling dental pain, there are practical advantages. When the patients are free from pain and anxiety, the dentist works more efficiently. And when the procedure is finished, neither patient nor dentist is exhausted.

At a pediatric clinical pharmacology meeting held at the National Institutes of Health in 1976, participants agreed that the situation "in the study of anesthetic agents, which would require a combination of competence in pediatrics, pharmacology, and anesthesiology was considered to be of critical dimensions." When the organizers of that meeting were asked what they planned to do to promote research in pediatric anesthetics in view of the concern expressed by the participants of that meeting, the reply was "Well, we held the meeting and published the report."

This attitude, common among the organizers of scientific meetings, always reminds me of a Mutt and Jeff comic strip I saw years ago. Mutt explains to Jeff his invention for preventing head-on collisions of trains: When the engineer sees a train coming at him on the same track, he releases a spring beneath his train that lifts it from the track. The oncoming train passes safely under it. "But," says Jeff, "what happens to the train in the air?" Says Mutt, "I've got nothing to do with the train once it leaves the tracks."

Not only is medicine prolonging the lives of people who have cancer, but also the burned, the maimed, the arthritics, the diabetics, and victims of strokes. The adults are becoming vocal. But suffering children have yet to find their spokesmen. As we have seen in this chapter, thousands of children suffer acute, chronic, and intermittent chronic pain from diseases, injuries, and diagnostic and treatment procedures. Enacted every day in hospitals are scenes in which children beg for pain relief, or put on a show of bravery to win approval from nurses and mothers and fathers. Or the child may writhe in agony, his suffering disregarded because an analgesic must be administered only according to schedule.

It is curious that mothers haven't risen to protest the unnecessary suffering of their children. Are they intimidated by the hospital system? Very likely. And there is the parents' fear of reprisal on the children if they complain too loudly. But mothers have been the moving spirits behind national organizations to combat diseases afflicting their children—hemophilia, leukemia, epilepsy, and many others. These women have not only organized agencies, but have raised millions of dollars to support them and have convinced congressmen to appropriate millions more. Surely in our time pain qualifies as a major disease in children. Where are the specialists in pediatric pain control? How many pediatric pain clinics are there in this country? None. They will come only when mothers and fathers demand that the

Congress appropriate funds for research and training for physicians, nurses, and psychologists in understanding and controlling physical and mental pain suffered by children.

8 the Pain Policy

Does your doctor like you?

How a doctor reacts to you as a person influences the medical care he gives you. Technically, the doctor gives the same quality care to all his patients. If a surgeon doesn't like you especially as a person, he will still cut you open as deftly as he cuts open a respected colleague. But, like everyone else, doctors have personal and social prejudices that openly or subtly influence their behavior with patients.

I doubt very much that former President Ford's wife was told she had breast cancer in quite the same way as was my hairdresser when she went to her doctor's office to find out the results of a biopsy test. Bluntly, her doctor told her she had cancer of the breast and that she was to report to the hospital on a certain date to have the breast removed.

He did not explain what the operation entailed, how extensive the surgery would be, whether it would impair the use of her arm and thereby affect her ability to earn her living as a hairdresser. Nor did he mention rehabilitation therapy. Shocked and utterly intimidated by his overbearing manner, she didn't ask any questions; but before and after the breast removal, she was in despair.

Months after the operation, she went back to hairdressing, her arm rehabilitated, but not her psyche.

The doctor-patient relationship is going through a traumatic period of adjustment as the beatified image of the healer fades into medical mythology. The art of medicine is being commercialized, mechanized, and impersonalized. Wistfully, older people look back on the days when a kindly, unhurried doctor braved blizzards and long distances to be at the bedside, dispensing comfort, relieving the patient's and the family's anxiety, leaving behind a sense of hope.

There have always been barriers to mutual understanding between doctors and patients, differences in education, social position, intelligence, whether a person was a "charity" patient or rich, religion, and national origins. But the breach has been widened in the last few decades as doctors serve more patients in less time and rely more on automated tests and mechanical devices for diagnosis and treatment.

The doctor-patient relationship varies with the two people involved. It may be formal, more like the relationship one has with a lawyer. Or it may be relaxed and friendly in the doctor's office and quite the opposite in the hospital where he is transfigured into a power figure, awesome to a helpless, dependent patient. As more women go into medical practice, relationships become more ambivalent, sex prejudices surfacing, quite frequently on the part of women themselves who "under no circumstances would consult a woman doctor."

Patients' attitudes swing from reverential at times to unreasonably demanding at others, treating the doctor as master one minute and servant the next. Most common has been the child-parent relationship in which the patient responds as the obedient child, eager to please by being a good patient, following instructions explicitly, never asking questions, giving the doctor absolute control. Once in a while, there is an adversary relationship. A sullen, distrustful patient leans back and silently challenges the doctor to cure him. And when doctor and patient do not speak a common language, the results can be confused and sometimes disastrous.

As, consumer attitudes permeate our society, the doctor-knows-best attitude is being steadily eroded. Public discontent shows up in malpractice suits, patients' rights manifestoes, group action complaints to hospital administrators, public indignation over unnecessary, costly diagnostic tests, letters of protest to newspaper editors, and heated panel discussions on television and radio. People who had not realized they had medical rights learn about them in newspaper accounts of court battles. A few courageous physicians, ignoring the wrath of colleagues, are publicly urging patients to get up off their knees.

As doctors are being pulled from their pedestals, there are a few points that should be considered. In the preface to his play, *The Doctor's Dilemma,* George Bernard Shaw said:

> For the strength of the doctor's, as of every other man's position when the evolution of social organization at last reaches his profession, will be that he will always have open to him the alternative of public employment when the private employer becomes too tyrannous. And let no one suppose that the words doctor and patient can disguise from the parties the fact that they are employer and employee. No doubt doctors who are in great demand can be as highhanded and independent as employees are in all classes when a dearth in their labor market makes them indispensable; but the average doctor is not in this position: he is struggling for life in an overcrowded profession. . . .

The private, solo practitioner is a medical freelance, his income dependent on the number of patients he treats. Hence, aptly termed "waiting rooms" resemble airline terminals in the Christmas season. If like airlines he "overbooks," one reason is that there are many "no show" patients. More people go to doctors now because medical and health insurance pay much of the cost. But the doctor's increased income is somewhat offset by the time he spends on forms and on untangling legal snarls with insurance and governmental agencies. To keep up with medical developments, he reads numerous journals, attends medical meetings, and takes continuing educational courses. Along with all that, he visits patients in hospitals and nursing homes, and, in extreme emergencies, makes house calls. He has little time left for the leisurely, compassionate healing that made his grandfather's doctor so beloved.

Before being licensed to practice, the physician goes through grueling years in medical school and two to three more years in hospital training. With that background, it is understandable if he or she does not have high regard for patients who do not know their pancreas from their liver and take better care of their cars than of their own bodies. If people were required to pass a simple physiology test before being accepted as patients, medical practice would go out of business.

It is, of course, much easier to be a passive patient than an informed medical client. It takes a certain nerve to look a physician in the eye and ask for explanations of alternatives to a prescribed treatment, or to ask for second or third medical opinions, or to refuse surgery. A 72-year-old man, debilitated by a chronic heart condition, meekly agreed to have a coronary bypass operation, spent eight hours on the operating table, and died there. Passivity accounts for the outrageous examples of people who have had twenty or more operations on their backs for chronic pain and who live in an analgesic bog.

But consumer activists are beginning to see medical care for what it is—America's third largest industry and the physician as a businessman in a white coat. And some doctors are taking the same point of view. In Washington, D.C., a group of doctors working for a prepaid health plan, salaried employees whose patient-members control the Group Health Associates, petitioned the National Labor Relations Board for recognition as a union.

In this climate, still very transitional, patients can speak up, request information about alternative types of treatment, and work out with their physicians long-term plans for dealing with chronic illness, including pain management. That is not to say that patients should march into the doctor's office carrying a copy of *The Merck Manual of Diagnosis and Therapy* (a marvelous reference book for the home hypochondriac) under one arm, but it does suggest that the activist patient should take more interest in his or her medical care. And in the long run, will get better care than the submissive biologically illiterate patient.

There would be fewer "anxious daughters," as physicians and nurses term worried women who plague them with complaints about the unrelieved suffering of parents in hospitals and nursing homes, if patients and members of their families asked questions at the onset of chronic illness. The physician who brilliantly handles emergencies, is uncanny in his diagnoses, who sets your broken wrist with skill and dispatch, whose clever hands stitched your son's forehead so no scar marked the place cut by a shattered windshield, may not have the skill or

the temperament for dealing with frustrating, unreward-
ing long-term care of cancer, arthritis, diabetes, or degenerative diseases of the bones.

Medical school training has not yet caught up with the
facts of medical needs, that there are two distinct types
of medical care needed today, acute and the chronic
with chronic disease far more prevalent. Before World
War II, 30 percent of all diseases were chronic; now 80
percent are. Doctors who expertly control acute, temporary pain, when confronted by pain they cannot diagnose or long-term pain, often fall back on a philosophical approach: "You'll just have to live with it." The
patient's response to that should be: "How?"

A doctor who cannot find the cause for persistent pain
in six months is not likely to find it in the next six months,
or in a year, or ever. If the only alternatives he offers are
powerful pain relievers or radical surgery, he is in a
sense already abandoning his patient: Powerful drugs
pacify patients and surgery shifts the problem to another doctor. The patient or the family should look for
another doctor who is equipped by training, experience,
temperament, and interest to deal with chronic pain of
known or unknown origins. Until recently, there were
no alternatives for desperate people except desperate
measures. But with the proliferation of pain clinics, patients can seek help before pain erodes their life force
and pain behavior puts down deep roots.

If pain is likely to develop in the course of a chronic
disease, the patient should ask the doctor what the pain
management plan will be, types of medications in the
early and later stages, and alternatives to drug therapy,
such as nerve blocks, biofeedback, psychotherapy. An
obvious but seldom asked question is the estimated
monthly cost of medication and treatment, especially
for people who are not old enough for Medicare.

A doctor may have a comprehensive plan for managing long-range pain, but may run into problems with the patient and the family. A Chicago physician, who for obvious reasons does not wish to be identified, says he has had patients who, though suffering from painful cancer, refused analgesics on religious grounds. Others had a need to suffer. And he has had a few instances in which embittered wives, particularly those whose husbands have been unfaithful, have told him: "Let the son of a bitch suffer!"

Doctors should prepare patients for the course pain is likely to take, the ebbing periods when medication should be reduced, especially the case with arthritic pain. Dr. Thomas McPherson Brown, director of the Arthritis Institute of the National Orthopedic Rehabilitation Hospital in Arlington, Virgina, says the medication helps for a time, then the body rejects it. "But if you leave it alone for a while, it begins to work again. In flare reactions, there is a cycle in which medication is blocked when the joint becomes acutely inflamed. Inflammation usually calms down on its own. If the dosage of the pain reliever is too high, the body begins to reject the medication. There are times when the arthritic can get along on very little medication and then in other phases of a cycle, larger doses are needed. Physicians should know those patterns for each patient and should adapt treatment accordingly."

In treating an arthritic, it sometimes occurs that a drug may in the beginning aggravate the condition through the mechanism of antigen release triggered by the medication, but later on the drug improves the condition. "If the physician knows from experience the likelihood of this pattern of aggravation followed by relief, and tells the patient what to expect, the patient will accept that flare-up without any problems," Dr. Brown says. "But if you don't explain that this pattern may be necessary before ultimate improvement is achieved, you will have an unnecessarily disturbed individual whose pain may be much worse because of psychological stress induced by lack of understanding. When people know the nature of a problem, it's amazing how well they can deal with it."

Knowing what is ahead enables patients to plan for it, financially and in other ways. For instance, the diagnosis of a chronic illness could influence a decision to change jobs or alter plans to retire to a distant place far from family and friends. But the time to discuss these matters with a doctor is in the early stages of the disease, not in the later crisis stage when sound decisions are hard to make, choices are reduced, and there is no time for putting affairs in order.

The physician's preferred route to medical care leads directly to the hospital, despite the fact that, once his patients get into the hospital care system, he loses a great deal of control over their treatment. His preference for the hospital rather than home care is based on his personal convenience, and the professional and legal advantages of the hospital. It's more convenient for a doctor to see several patients in one place. The hospital gives him limitless technical resources and a backup of specialists. The hospital's accounting department relieves him of much paperwork by taking care of the mechanics of "third-party" payments. And, in the edgy climate of malpractice suits, forced now to practice defensive medicine, doctors feel more secure legally when their patients are in a hospital. If a patient who has had a heart attack dies in a hospital coronary unit, the doctor is less vulnerable legally than he might be had he not sent the patient to the hospital, even though the attack may have seemed slight.

The hospital provides other professional advantages. It is a place where doctors get together to discuss cases and their presence in the hospital gives them a certain visibility that enhances their professional standing with each other. Even being paged over the hospital public address system adds a few prestige points.

From the doctor's viewpoint, then, the hospital has all sorts of advantages for him, but for patients with long-term illness the advantages are getting harder to identify. No one questions the value of hospital emergency rooms, the critical care units, outpatient department, surgical and obstetrical services, and the innovative in-and-out-the-same-day surgical units. But as a place for treating the chronically ill, the hospital is an anachronism. About one-third to one-half of patients in hospitals really don't belong there; their condition does not justify the highly trained personnel and the sophisticated equipment. Under the guise of paying for room, meals, nursing, and other services, patients are paying the exorbitant costs of automated clinical laboratory systems, electronic diagnostic machines (in some hospitals $600,-000 scanners), computer systems, research laboratories, elaborate life-sustaining equipment, and monitors.

Originally, hospitals were pest houses, places for the very poor, derelicts, and gravely ill or injured sailors who used to be carried off ships at night and dumped on the doorsteps of houses near the docks. It was whispered among the poor that whoever went into the hospital never came out again, dead or alive, for they kept the bodies and cut them up. Respectable families took care of their own at home.

Now, by a curious kind of regression, hospitals once again engender uneasiness in the public mind, hazardous places where infections abound, horrendous diagnostic tests, inept treatment, and a shocking number of fatal drug interactions. People are turning back to the home as the safest, most comfortable and economical place of primary care.

But now it's a different kind of home care. Trained professionals and volunteers play roles once played by parents, brothers and sisters, and aunts and uncles. The Health Insurance Institute reports a trend toward home-care coverage in individual and group health insurance policies. Some large industries include home-care benefits in employee medical insurance. Employees of the Eastman Kodak Company, for one, are covered for up to 90 days of home health care a year. Under this plan, hospital stays have been reduced by as much as 21 days a patient. Profit-making firms such as Homemakers Upjohn and voluntary and local governmental agencies offer a range of services—housekeeping, nursing, therapy.

Whereas pain management in a hospital is peripheral to the treatment of the disease, in a home-care program it is an intrinsic part of care. At home, a person has more control of his treatment and therapy. One who would be bedbound in a hospital might very well get up and walk about at home, do things for himself, and, with family help, practice his personal version of operant conditioning. Families are spared trips to the hospital at inconvenient hours and in all weather, the stress of limited privacy in visiting, and anxiety over the patient's obvious, unrelieved suffering. Under the supervision of a physician or nurse, chronic or terminal pain can be better managed in the home than in the hospital where it is no one's responsibility.

When Dr. Maurice B. Strauss, former professor at Tufts University Medical School, knew after irradiation had failed to control his cancer that he would die, he was determined to spend his remaining days in the familiar and satisfying setting of his home. Shortly before he died, two of his former students, Dr. Walter Hollander, Jr., and Dr. R. Franklin Williams visited their beloved teacher and later wrote about that visit in an article, "Dr. Strauss' Last Teaching Lesson."[1]

In regard to the control of pain, Dr. Strauss told his visitors that in the early course of the disease, he had delayed taking opiates until his pain became moderately severe. But he found that each new dose took too long to work. Within an hour or so, the pain became even more severe, requiring another injection that still did not give enough relief. He changed the schedule so that he received morphine routinely every four hours by the clock, which prevented the pain without noticeably depressive side effects. Here was a professor of medicine who, first, chose home rather than the hospital and then used trial and error until he found a pain control method that worked for him.

This would be true for most any patient at home. And at home, one at least in which a harmonious relationship exists, the perception of pain would be modified by the familiar surroundings and the absence of hospital stress. In a study[2] of hospital stress factors, among the forty-nine items described as sources of psychosocial stress for hospital patients the fear of not getting relief from pain medications, and not getting the pain medication when needed, ranked among the highest perceived stresses.

In his message to Congress on his administration's first health initiatives, President Carter said, "Debt from hospitalization is the leading cause of personal bankruptcy in the United States." He went on to say that excessive spending by hospitals produces worse, not better care. "When unnecessary procedures are performed, the patient is subjected to needless risk of injury or death."

Considering the evidence that hospitals are neither the most effective nor the safest places for patients, why has there not been more federal support for home-care programs? One reason is bureaucratic resistance. It is easier to administer the reimbursement of medical costs through the hospital system. Covertly, federal officials exert powerful influence over legislation. Congressional staff aides, hungry for legislative suggestions, too pressed to research every subject for the many bills congressmen introduce to keep their legislative status viable, depend on agency officials for ideas. In this way, governmental officials who would be obliged to administer certain legislated programs influence their fate. Some of these officials have successfully convinced congressional staff aides that home-care programs are a muddle to administer. Indirectly, this attitude perpetuates the hospital-care system as the only alternative because it is tightly organized and much easier to work with in keeping tabs on services and reimbursements.

But word from constituents is seeping through congressional pipelines about the need for home-care services, especially for the chronically ill. In the first few weeks of 1977, congressmen had already sponsored 13 bills on home care. One, sponsored by Senator Edward W. Brooke of Massachusetts, would eliminate the required three-day hospital stay before a person would be eligible for Medicare payments for home care, a seemingly small matter, but one that has enormous implications for millions of people.

As more health insurance policyholders request home-care coverage, the faster supporting services will be developed. More nurses, housekeepers, and paid therapists to help people remain in their homes will bring about a twentieth-century version of the care formerly given in the home by members of large families and concerned neighbors.

Grave debilitating illness that foreshortens life and creates special pain management problems cannot always be handled at home, especially if a person lives alone or is dependent on a relative who cannot cope with the constant care and worry. In such cases, the alternative may be a nursing home, a difficult emotional decision for families to make, and a crushing financial burden.

Dr. Arthur Levin, in *Talk Back to Your Doctor,* his book addressed to the new type of medical client and covering every aspect of medical care, says, "Nursing homes are dangerous places. Too often sending someone to a nursing home is the same as signing their death certificate." But if there is no alternative, he advises families to visit several nursing homes, looking over kitchens, baths, physical and occupational therapy sections, and checking on the ratio of nurses to patients, provisions for physician care, dietary and dental care, recreational and spiritual activities. If the home is too quiet, it may be a sign that all patients are drugged into a stupor. "Use your nose," he advises. "The smell of urine or feces can mean only one thing: somewhere a patient is lying in them."

Before entering a relative in a nursing home, the family should discuss the pain control program with the administrator. A policy of giving analgesics only when patients in severe pain ask for them guarantees trouble. Pain medication should be given on a regular basis as it is in hospices, the dose adjusted to the patient and his pain problem, and administered on a schedule that ensures keeping ahead of the pain without putting the patient into a semi-comatose state.

If the pain policy were discussed beforehand, there would be fewer "anxious daughters" complaining about the needless suffering of parents, writing letters to their congressmen and to governmental officials, begging them to do something about the suffering of a parent in a particular nursing home. All that anguish could have been prevented had daughter or son, husband or wife, taken a stand at the outset, backed by the family physician. Fear of reprisals on the patient should not deter the family. Nursing homes are run for profit, many of them units in national hotel chain companies whose stocks are listed on the stock exchange and whose managers are sensitive to bad publicity. Nor do they wish to see government inspectors arriving unexpectedly. Periodic visits by the family doctor further bolster the patient's status and morale and let the nursing home director and the staff know that the patient has not been medically abandoned.

Those who strive to remain outside hospitals and nursing homes are finding ways of coping with pain through self-help groups. One such group is Chronic Pain Outreach, started in 1976 by Gwendolyn Talbot, a speech pathologist in Manassas, Virginia. Members of the group suffer from many types of chronic pain, including disk deterioration, bone and muscle pain from accidents, headaches, pain resulting from surgery, arthritis, cancer, stroke, and other causes.

More than a hand-holding group, it gives its members an understanding of the options of controlling their pain and information about resources within the state and nearby Washington, D.C., area. Members are told their rights as patients and encouraged to take a stand for them. When one member of the group told them her doctor had diagnosed her condition as "M.S." and had not explained what the initials stood for, she was berated by the group for not asking him.

The members of this group rate themselves on a one-to-ten scale of pain intensity, noting differences in the perception of pain under emotional stress, learning that, though the nature of the pain does not change, their reactions to it do. Family members attend sessions to learn how to cope with the pain situation, what they may be doing that prevents a wife or a husband from coping better, and what positive behavior they should adopt.

"The group members," says Gwendolyn Talbot, "are not looking for sympathy. They want to talk with others who 'know where they are at,' who understand not only the vagaries of chronic pain and its tidal effects, but how to help each other with insights into the influences that change pain perception. And some want practical advice on such matters as how to enjoy sex despite a painful disability."

Members of the group, which meets twice a month, are in varying states of pain. Some have total remission for a time. As word about the group spread through the area, physicians began referring to the group patients they can no longer help. "We hope eventually to be associated with a pain clinic," Miss Talbot says, "remaining a separate voluntary group, but one in which those who have completed a pain control series of treatment would have support in maintaining the treatment, continuing exercises, keeping on special diets, practicing biofeedback, or whatever continuing responsibility the person has for maintaining pain control."[8]

Concurrent with the self-help movement is medical self-care pioneered by Dr. Keith Sehnert of Georgetown University. Author of *How to Be Your Own Doctor—*

Sometimes, Dr. Sehnert has conducted training courses for nonprofessionals throughout the country. The training teaches people to monitor their own health, screen themselves for early signs of illness, treat minor ailments, and cut down on unnecessary calls on the doctor. By being informed about common medical problems and responsible for his or her health, the trained person becomes the primary member of the coordinated health care team.

The new medical self-care movement has caught on with thousands of nonprofessionals, business people, housewives, retired workers, and some physicians. Like any new movement, it has its enthusiastic advocates and detractors, among the latter physicians who see it as a threat and fraught with dire consequences. An ardent advocate is Tom Ferguson who, while a medical student at Yale University, gave training courses himself, then launched the magazine *Medical Self-Care*[4] that quickly attracted thousands of readers. In the Winter 1977/78 issue, he set forth the principles of the medical self-care movement:

> Most lay people know far too little about evaluating and improving their health *without* waiting until they get sick, and about coping with illness—both through self-care and by making good use of health care facilities—when illness does occur. The Self-Care movement feels that we have depended too much on experts in health care; that with the proper training and self-study materials, lay people would be capable of being their own paramedics.

For chronic pain sufferers, pain clinics, self-help groups, and medical self-care offer dynamic alternatives to passive acceptance of pain-caused disability and marginal lives.

President Carter's edict regarding the testing of all

drugs, including heroin, marijuana, and LSD, for their possible use in controlling terminal cancer pain was the first high-level recognition of cancer pain as a widespread problem. But the testing of these drugs for use in one type of pain is only one small step toward alleviating suffering. A broad attack on the pain epidemic that would include coordinated research, training, evaluation of current pain control methods, and physician and public education in the myriad treatment alternatives requires congressional interest and backing. It is the Congress that sanctions health programs and authorizes the money to pay for them. Without congressional mandates and funds, President Carter's initiative could fizzle out in that bog of the bureaucratic substitute for action —committees, meetings, and conferences, long-range plans that never get implemented, "front office" reports that nobody reads.

Congressmen cannot keep up with every aspect of health, energy, foreign trade, inflation, crime, national security, the arms race, unemployment, detente, and all the other subjects that are inextricably part of American life. Congressmen depend on experts within and outside the government, on special interest groups, and on individual constituents to inform them about problems and suggest ideas for legislation.

The general feeling that individuals can do little to influence the Congress is unfounded. It is a matter of knowing how to go about it—the techniques of influence. Most skillful at this are the professional influencers, the Washington lobbyists or, as they prefer to call themselves, congressional liaisons, representing special interests who track legislation in the Congress, attend hearings on bills, know what is in the legislative pipeline and when bills will be voted on in the House and Senate. Registered lobbyists, outnumbering congressmen by the hundreds, are not, as is commonly supposed, only those representing commercial interests. There are lobbyists for consumers, the environment, nurses, the handicapped, organizations for and against abortion, and minority rights; just about any interest one could think of has its lobbyists in Washington.

Besides the professional lobbyists there are those who might be termed successful amateurs. Mary Lasker, America's public health matriarch, a rich, formerly successful business woman, has influenced more major health legislation than most public officials. As an ardent public health proponent, she was behind the establishment of the National Heart and Lung Institute, national mental health programs, the high blood pressure education program, and the national research program in anesthesiology. It was she who persuaded chairmen of congressional appropriations committees to invite health experts from outside the government to testify at budget hearings. And the Lasker Awards are among the most prestigious in medical science.

Another private citizen expert in influencing the Congress is Jules Stein, at one time a professional musician and an ophthalmologist, head of the Music Corporation of America. He rallied heavy professional support among ophthalmologists with the result that the Congress authorized the National Eye Institute in 1970, the primary eye research institute in America.

Florence Mahoney, widow of a former newspaper editor, spent years urging members of the Congress to authorize a national institute on aging. The Congress finally passed the bill, but President Nixon vetoed it. Undaunted, Florence Mahoney went at it again, pressed on, and, in 1974, the National Institute on Aging was established.

After folksinger Woodie Guthrie died of Huntington's

chorea, a rare, mentally and physically devastating genetic disease, his widow, Margerie, began a crusade for research on the disease. She badgered officials of the National Institutes of Health into providing funds for a national commission and persuaded Congressman Robert Roe to introduce a bill to amend the Public Health Service Act to provide assistance for programs for diagnosis, prevention, and research in Huntington's chorea.

The identity of the moving spirit behind a bold congressional or White House action is sometimes lost in the excitement of headlines and official consternation. Without in any way detracting from Dr. Peter Bourne's political courage in gaining President Carter's approval for the directive to reassess heroin and other drugs for medicinal purposes, it should be pointed out that the moving spirit behind that controversial action was a private citizen, Judith Quattlebaum. Since 1976 when she organized the National Committee on the Treatment of Intractable Pain, she crusaded in the press and in the Congress for a change in the federal policy prohibiting the medicinal use of heroin.

Mrs. Quattlebaum sent a series of letters and sustaining evidence to her congressman, Newton I. Steers, Jr., of Maryland, about the plight of terminal cancer patients and the need for the government to make heroin available to physicians for treating intractable pain. Congressman Steers forwarded her letters to Congressman Paul Rogers of Florida (referred to on Capitol Hill as "Mr. Health"), chairman of the Subcommittee on Health and the Environment, who in turn sent them to Dr. Bourne. Dr. Bourne, whose personal sentiments inclined him to favoring studies of heroin and other proscribed drugs for medicinal benefits, and backed by the two powerful congressmen, took up the matter with President Carter and obtained his approval for the directive.

Anyone who doubts the power of the dedicated, persistent private citizen to influence the Congress or the White House should use the name of Judith Quattlebaum to erase those doubts.

As late as 1977, the Congress had not heard from public or voluntary agency health officials about the magnitude of the pain problem in America, the millions of afflicted Americans young and old, and the billions it costs in medical care and disability payments. Each year the number afflicted escalates—disabling injuries in highway accidents and industry; new cases of cancer, stroke, and arthritis; degenerative bone disease; more men, women, and children undergoing continuous diagnostic and treatment procedures for chronic ailments; and the suffering children whose lives have been salvaged by new medical techniques. Only one group has benefited handsomely from the government's neglect of pain research and treatment and that is the quacks.

That federal public health officials have ignored this overwhelming problem can be attributed only to the fact that national health priorities are determined by a mixture of caprice and political expedience. When a new president is elected, old-line public health officials ask each other, "Well, what ails *him*?" Whatever it is, there is a rush to the laboratories to investigate it.

In the present self-help climate, medical consumers can do something to influence the Congress. Congressmen pay attention to letters from constituents when those letters indicate that the writer knows what he is talking about either from personal or professional experience. Harley Dirks, former staff aide to the Senate Appropriations Committee, an experienced reader of letters from constituents, says that the letters of grassroots lobbyists get attention. His advice is to keep them to one page—handwritten or typed—stating straight off what the subject is, followed by an explanation of the problem, backed by facts about its magnitude, the human and money costs, a brief personal example if it adds emphasis and drama to the facts, and ending with specific suggestions for what should be done.

Appropriate allies to enlist for action on the pain problem are physicians, heads of local medical societies, chairmen of voluntary health agencies, and directors of rehabilitation centers who know the cost of pain in disability payments. Keenly interested in the subject of pain control, well aware of the need for research on better analgesics are dentists, who would benefit in every way from new, safer, more effective pain relievers. Medical and health insurance companies, ever on the alert for ways of reducing hospital and disability costs, have a financial stake in pain control programs and, through their sophisticated lobbyists, have considerable congressional influence.

Other sources of advocates are consumer groups, and medical directors of labor unions and industrial plants. Among lobbyists, who by law are required to register their special interests with the Congress, are many primarily concerned with health. For the public good and to burnish their own public image, some of these lobbyists could be persuaded to support legislation aimed at mounting a national pain control program. (See page 212 for list of registered health lobbyists.)

You do not need an M.D. or Ph.D. degree to qualify as an expert. Congressman Jim Wright in his book *You and Your Congressman* says, "Not every citizen can influence the course of history in a major way. But those who wish to do so, depending upon the individual will and perseverance, definitely can make their opinions felt in high places of government. Occasionally, since ours is the kind of government it is, one private individual actually can create a chain reaction which will result in a truly broad and meaningful national policy."

The purpose of a grass-roots lobbying effort for a national pain program is to convince Congress of the need for action by the Public Health Service, a program that would not require special funds, but a realignment of health priorities in which the pain problem would be taken off the bottom rung and put close to the top where it belongs.

Americans are very vocal about how their tax dollars are spent but singularly indifferent to what voluntary agencies do with the money they collect. The sacrosanct aura surrounding nonprofit health agencies discourages contributors from asking questions or from suggesting how they wish their money to be spent. Yet each contributor is in a sense a stockholder. In business, stockholders expect to make money on their investment. What do contributors expect?

Do you really believe your money will buy a cure for cancer or for arthritis? A blind friend once told me that people give to blind beggars not out of compassion, but from superstitious fear that if they do not put a coin in the tin cup, evil spirits might afflict them with blindness. When you come down to it, much of our so-called philanthropy is motivated by that same visceral fear. But while placating the gods and warding off evil spirits, we could get more for our money than chancy protection against evil fate if we showed more interest in how our contributions are spent.

If for instance every potential contributor to the American Cancer Society and to the Arthritis Foundation, as a condition for contributing money, asked for a statement on what those agencies, concerned as they are with diseases in which pain is inherent, are doing in the field of pain control. Neither agency has supported pain control research, but if contributors showed an interest in the subject, there would be an upsurge of agency activity in pain research, physician and nurse education in pain management, and possibly some specialized clinics for the treatment of cancer and arthritic pain. Unless contributors speak up, the problem will continue to be ignored because as a fund raiser the subject of pain does not set the blood racing.

Dr. Theodore Cooper, former Surgeon General, says that in fifty years we will die of the same diseases we die from now but, in the meantime, we'll be more comfortable. If the medical care for which we pay so dearly cannot cure us, at the very least it can ensure a mitigation of distress by the relief of pain.

And George Bernard Shaw said:

> Use your health, even to the point of wearing it out. That is what it is for. Spend all you have before you die; and do not outlive yourself.

CHAPTER NOTES

CHAPTER ONE
1. James E. Turner, "I'm fed up with research sensationalism!" *Medical Economics,* January 20, 1969, 215–224.
2. Source: Edward Jay Epstein, *Agency of Fear: Opiates and Political Power in America,* 1977, 86–92.

CHAPTER TWO
1. C. Norman Shealy with Arthur S. Freese, *Occult Medicine Can Save Your Life,* 1975, 177.
2. Sources for the brief statements of religious concepts are: *Jewish Medical Ethics* by Dr. Immanuel Jakobovits; Dr. Dikwela Piyananda of the Buddhist Vihara Society of Washington, D.C.; Dr. Muhammad Abdul Rauf, Islamic Center, Washington, D.C.; Rev. Daniel Gatti, S.J., Georgetown University Hospital, and other members of the clergy; and H. Dickinson Rathbun, Christian Science Office, Washington, D.C.
3. Richard A. Sternbach, *Pain Patients: Traits and Treatment,* 1974, 10 & 11.
4. Dorothy Clarke Wilson, *Ten Fingers for God,* 1965, 142–145.

CHAPTER THREE
1. F. J. Ingelfinger, "Cancer! Alarm! Cancer!" *New England Journal of Medicine,* December 18, 1975, 1319 & 1320.
2. Mark Mehta, *Intractable Pain,* 1973, 130 & 131.
3. Excerpt from an address by Dr. Robert G. Twycross at the meeting of the National Committee on the Treatment of Intractable Pain, Washington, D.C., January 31, 1978. The full text of Dr. Twycross's address may be obtained from the National Committee on the Treatment of Intractable Pain, P.O. Box 34571, Washington, D.C. 20034.
4. S. E. Sallan, N. E. Zinberg, and E. Frei, III, "Antiemetic Effect of Delta-9-Tetrahydrocannabinol in Patients Receiving Cancer Chemotherapy," *New England Journal of Medicine,* October 16, 1975, 795–797.
5. Source: Stephen K. Carter and Lorraine M. Kershner, "What You Should Know about Drugs vs. Cancer," *Pharmacy Times,* August 1975, 56–66.
6. For information about hospices in the United States write: National Hospice Organization, c/o Hospice, Inc., 765 Prospect St., New Haven, Connecticut 06511.

CHAPTER FOUR

For the title of this chapter, "Painmanship," I am indebted to Dr. Thomas S. Szasz who coined the term.

1. Carl M. Grossman and Sylva Grossman, *The Wild Analyst: Life and Work of Georg Groddeck,* 1965, 80 & 81.
2. I. Pilowsky, "The Psychiatrist and the Pain Clinic," *American Journal of Psychiatry,* July 1976, 755.
3. Eric Berne, *Games People Play,* 1964, 85–87.

CHAPTER FIVE

1. Dr. Jane spoke at a seminar on pain organized by the Society for Neuroscience for science writers. It was at this meeting that Harold M. Schmeck, Jr., of the *New York Times* and other journalists on a panel tried to explain to the scientists why newspaper editors rarely feel as excited about basic research as those who do it.
2. Ronald Melzack, "The Gate Theory Revisited," *Current Concepts in the Management of Chronic Plain,* Pierre L. LeRoy, editor, 1977, 79–92.

CHAPTER SIX

1. A. Strauss, S. Y. Fagerhaugh, and B. Glaser, "Pain: An Organizational-Work-Interactional Perspective," *Nursing Outlook,* September 1974, 560–566.
2. Thomas P. Hackett, "Pain and Prejudice," *Medical Times,* February 1971, 134.
3. Bernard E. Finneson with Arthur S. Freese, *Dr. Finneson on Low Back Pain,* 1975, 46–51.
4. Carolyn L. Wiener, "Pain Assessment on an Orthopedic Ward," *Nursing Outlook,* August 1975, 508–516.
5. Two of these studies have been cited. The third, which deserves equal attention, is by S. Y. Fagerhaugh, "Pain Expression and Control on a Burn Care Unit," *Nursing Outlook,* October 1974, 645–650.
6. Wilbert E. Fordyce, *Behavioral Methods for Chronic Pain and Illness,* 1976, 144 & 145.
7. Barbara B. Brown, *New Mind, New Body: Bio-Feedback: New Directions for the Mind,* 1975. A fascinating account of the development of biofeedback.
8. Excerpts from an interview with Dr. Harold J. Wain on American University's radio station WAMU-FM, January 20, 1977.

9. Copies of the directory may be purchased from: Executive Office, American Society of Anesthesiologists, 515 Busse Highway, Park Ridge, Illinois 60068.
10. Richard A. Sternbach, op. cit., 92.
11. Linda D. Winslow, "Pain, Part II, A Personalized Approach," *Journal of Practical Nursing*, February 1977, 16–17, 34 & 41.

CHAPTER SEVEN
1. Nancy V. Schultz, "How Children Perceive Pain," *Nursing Outlook*, October 1971, 670–673.
2. Norman R. Bernstein, *Emotional Care of the Facially Burned and Disfigured*, 1976, 134–136.
3. Margo McCaffery, "Pain Relief for the Child," *Pediatric Nursing*, July–August 1977, 11–16.
4. *Pediatric Clinical Pharmacology*, report on workshop, November 18–19, 1976, Bethesda, Maryland [DHEW Publication No. (NIH) 77–1282].

CHAPTER EIGHT
1. Walter Hollander, Jr., and T. Franklin Williams, "Dr. Strauss' Last Teaching Session," *Archives of Internal Medicine*, 135:1391, pages 62–64.
2. B. J. Volicer, M. A. Isenberg, and M. W. Burns, "Medical-Surgical Differences in Hospital Stress Factors," *Journal of Human Stress*, June 1977, 7.
3. For more information about Chronic Pain Outreach write to: Gwendolyn Talbot, 8222 Wycliffe Court, Manassas, Virginia 22110 (Phone: 703 368-7357).
4. Subscriptions to *Medical Self-Care* may be obtained from: *Medical Self-Care*, Box 717, Inverness, California 94937.

BIBLIOGRAPHY

Articles and books cited under "Chapter Notes" are more fully identified in this list, which also includes additional background reading.

Ackerman, L. V., and del Regato, J. *Cancer: Diagnosis, Treatment, and Prognosis.* Fourth Edition. St. Louis, C. V. Mosby Co., 1970.

Arias, J. "Christ Has No Love for Pain." *The Sign,* July–August 1976.

Berne, E. *Games People Play.* New York, Grove Press, 1964.

Bernstein, N. R. *Emotional Care of Facially Burned and Disfigured.* Boston, Little, Brown, 1976.

Bonica, J. J. *The Management of Pain.* Philadelphia, Lea & Febiger, 1954.

Bonica, J. J. (Ed.) *Advances in Neurology: Pain.* New York, Raven Press, 1974.

Bonica, J. J., and Albe-Fessard, D. *Advances in Pain Research and Therapy* (Proceedings of First World Congress on Pain). New York, Raven Press, 1976.

Brecher, E. and Editors of Consumer Reports. *Licit and Illicit Drugs.* Boston, Little, Brown and Co., 1972.

Brown, B. B. *New Mind, New Body: Bio-Feedback: New Directions for the Mind.* New York, Harper & Row, 1975.

Coleman, V. *The Medicine Men.* London, Temple Smith, 1975.

Copp, L. *The Pain Experience.* New York, McGraw-Hill, 1977.

De Quincey, T. *Confessions of an English Opium Eater,* with an introduction by William Bolitho. New York, The Heritage Press, 1950.

Dimond, E. G. *More than Herbs and Acupuncture.* New York, W. W. Norton & Co., Inc., 1975.

Duranty, W. *I Write As I Please.* New York, Simon and Schuster, 1935.

Efron, D. H. (Ed.) *Ethnopharmacologic Search for Psychoactive Drugs.* Washington, D.C., 1967 (Public Health Services Publication No. 1645).

Epstein, E. J. *Agency of Fear: Opiates and Political Power in America.* New York, G. P. Putnam's Sons, 1977.

Fagerhaugh, S. Y. "Pain Expression and Control on a Burn Care Unit." *Nursing Outlook,* Vol. 22, No. 10, October 1974.

Finneson, B. E., and Freese, A. S. *Dr. Finneson on Low Back Pain.* New York, G. P. Putnam's Sons, 1975.

Fordyce, W. E. *Behavioral Methods for Chronic Pain and Illness.* St. Louis, C. V. Mosby Co., 1976.

Freese, A. S. *Pain.* New York, G. P. Putnam's Sons, 1974.

Freud, A. "The Role of Bodily Illness in the Mental Life of Children." *The Psychoanalytic Study of the Child,* Vol. 7, 1952.

Glick, J. H. "A Doctor Prescribes Mercy." *Good Housekeeping,* August 1975.

Graham, H. *The Story of Surgery.* New York, Dorama & Co., 1939.

Grossman, C. M., and Grossman, S. *The Wild Analyst: The Life and Work of Georg Groddeck.* London, Barrie and Rockliff, 1965.

Guirdham, A. *A Theory of Disease.* London, Neville Spearman, Ltd., 1957.

Hackett, T. P. "Pain and Prejudice." *Medical Times,* Vol. 99, No. 2, February 1976.

Haggard, H. W. *Devils, Drugs, and Doctors.* New York, Harper & Brothers, 1929.

Hilgard, E. R., and Hilgard, J. R. *Hypnosis in the Relief of Pain.* Los Altos, California, William Kaufman, Inc., 1975.

Hospitalized Children. Bibliography 1976. Association for the Care of Children in Hospitals, P.O. Box H, Union, West Virginia.

Illich, I. *Medical Nemesis.* London. Calder & Boyers, 1975.

Jakobovits, I. *Jewish Medical Ethics.* New York, Block Publishing Co., 1959.

Jones, E. *The Life and Work of Sigmund Freud.* New York, Basic Books, 1957.

Keats, A. S. *New Concepts in Pain and Its Clinical Management.* Philadelphia, F. A. Davis Co., 1967.

Kirstein, G. G. *Better Giving.* Boston, Houghton Mifflin Co., 1975.

Koestler, A. *The Call Girls.* New York, Random House, 1973.

Lansky, S. "School Phobia in Children with Malignant Neoplasms." *American Journal of Diseases of Children,* Vol. 129, January 1975.

Leff, David. "Management of Chronic Pain: Medicine's New Growth Industry." *Medical World News,* October 18, 1976.

Leriche, René. *La Chirurgie de la Douleur.* Paris, Masson et cie, 1949.

LeRoy, P. L. (Ed.) *Current Concepts in the Management of Chronic Pain.* Miami, Symposia Specialists, 1977.

LeShan, L. *How to Meditate.* Boston, Little, Brown and Co., 1974.

LeShan, L. *You Can Fight for Your Life*. New York, M. Evans and Co., 1977.

Leventhal, B. G., and Hersh, S. "Modern Treatment of Childhood Leukemia." *Children Today*, May–June 1974.

Levin, A. *Talk Back to Your Doctor*. Garden City, N.Y., Doubleday & Co., 1975.

Lewis, C. S. *The Problem of Pain*. New York, Macmillan Co., 1943.

Major, R. H. *A History of Medicine*. Springfield, Mass., Charles C. Thomas, 1954.

Mandell, A. J. *The Nightmare Season*. New York, Random House, 1976.

McBride, M. M. "Assessing Children with Pain: Can You Tell Me Where It Hurts?" *Pediatric Nursing*, Vol. 3, No. 4, July–August 1977.

McCaffery, M. "Pain Relief for the Child." *Pediatric Nursing*, Vol. 3, No. 4, July–August 1977.

Mehta, M. *Intractable Pain*. London, W. B. Saunders Co., 1973.

Melzack, R. *The Puzzle of Pain*, New York, Basic Books, 1974.

Melzack, R., and Wall, P. D. "Pain Mechanisms: A New Theory." *Science*, Vol. 150, No. 3699, November 19, 1965.

Neal, H. (Ed.) *Better Communications for Better Health*. New York, Columbia University Press, 1962.

O'Rourke, K. D. (Ed.) *The Mission of Healing*. St. Louis, The Catholic Hospital Association, 1974.

Orwell, G. "How the Poor Die," *Collected Essays*. London, Secker & Warburg, 1961.

Pain. (brochure) Washington, D.C., 1968 (Public Health Service Publication No. 307–707).

Pediatric Clinical Pharmacology. Report on Workshop, November 18–19, 1976, Bethesda, Md. [DHEW Publication No. (NIH) 77-1282].

Petrie, A. *Individuality in Pain and Suffering*. Chicago, University Press, 1967.

Petrillo, M., and Sanger, S. *Emotional Care of Hospitalized Children*. New York, Lippincott, 1972.

Pilowsky, I. "The Psychiatrist and the Pain Clinic." *American Journal of Psychiatry*, 133:7, July 1976.

Proudfoot, M. *Suffering: A Christian Understanding*. Philadelphia, The Westminster Press, 1964.

Rettig, R. A. *Cancer Crusade*. Princeton, New Jersey, Princeton University Press, 1977.

Risley, M. *The House of Healing.* Garden City, N.Y., Doubleday and Co., 1961.

Rushmer, R. F. *Humanizing Health Care.* Cambridge, Mass., MIT Press, 1975.

Schultz, N. "How Children Perceive Pain." *Nursing Outlook,* Vol. 19, No. 10, October 1971.

Shaw, G. B. *Prefaces by Bernard Shaw* (Preface to *The Doctor's Dilemma*). London, Constable and Co., 1934.

Shealy, C. N., with Freese, A. S. *Occult Medicine Can Save Your Life.* New York, The Dial Press, 1975.

Sternbach, R. A. *Pain Patients: Traits and Treatment.* New York, Academic Press, 1974.

Strauss, A., Fagerhaugh, S. Y., and Glaser, B. "Pain: An Organizational-Work-Interactional Perspective." *Nursing Outlook,* Vol. 22, No. 9, September 1974.

Szasz, T. S. *Pain and Pleasure.* New York, Basic Books, Inc., 1957.

Szasz, T. S. *Ceremonial Chemistry.* Garden City, N.Y., Anchor Press/Doubleday, 1974.

Taubenhaus, M. *The Rights of Patients.* New York, Public Affairs Pamphlets, 1976.

Travell, J. *Office Hours: Day and Night.* Cleveland, Ohio, New American Library in association with The World Publishing Co., 1968.

Udall, M. K. *The Job of the Congressman.* Indianapolis, Bobbs-Merrill, 1970.

Vickery, D. M., and Fries, J. F. *Take Care of Yourself: A Consumer's Guide to Medical Care.* Reading, Mass., Addison-Wesley Publishing Co., 1976.

Weisenberg, M. (Ed.) *Pain: Clinical and Experimental Perspectives.* St. Louis, C. V. Mosby Co., 1975.

Wiener, C. L. "Pain Assessment on an Orthopedic Ward." *Nursing Outlook,* Vol. 23, No. 8, August 1975.

Wilson, D. C. *Ten Fingers for God.* New York, McGraw-Hill, 1965.

Woolmer, R. *The Conquest of Pain.* New York, Alfred A. Knopf, 1961.

Wright, J. *You and Your Congressman.* New York, Coward-McCann, 1965.

Zweig, S. *Mental Healers.* Garden City, N.Y., Garden City Publishing Co., 1931.

ACKNOWLEDGMENTS

Writing a book of this nature would have been impossible without the extraordinary cooperation of men and women inside and outside the medical and scientific professions. Many of them are physicians, nurses, scientists, psychologists, and social workers whom I quote and identify. But there are others who, dependent on federal grant funds or because of the strictures of their professional affiliations, preferred not to be identified with their comments on the political aspects of pain, but encouraged me to speak out. To all my sources within the medical and scientific professions who generously gave of their time to discuss myriad aspects of pain, my heartfelt thanks.

I am immensely indebted to Marc Stern, former colleague in the NIH Office of Communications, who for years conducted a sort of "pain alert" that kept me informed of articles, books, lectures, and meetings related to pain.

To Bowen Hosford, head of the NIH Audio-visual section, my thanks for coaching me in the techniques of radio interviewing and sanctioning the series of interviews I conducted with NIH scientists and administrators. Much of the information used in this book is based on those radio interviews.

After frustrating attempts to get information about pediatric pain—one of the most neglected areas in the whole field of pain —it was June L. McCalla, pediatric nurse specialist at the NIH Clinical Center, who gave me invaluable source materials and opened the way to further research on the subject. Another very helpful woman in this area was Grace Monaco, president of Candlelighters, the national organization of mothers of leukemic children.

One of the most gratifying things about writing this book was the network of friends who, "sensitized" by my interest in pain, clipped and sent me every printed reference to pain they came across. Wanda Warddell, my former associate at NIH and close personal friend, heads the list of those who never let a printed mention of pain slip by without spearing it for my files. Special thanks are also due my friends Vivian Dickson, Esther Gilbert, my sister-in-law Ida Neal, Naomi Thompson, and Katharine Toll for contributing unique bits of information. And to the professional researchers Nora Jean Levin, Daniel Nossiter, and Janet Steiger, my appreciation for tracking down data unavailable in published

210

materials. To my niece Patricia Emsellman, my gratitude for her encouragement and help.

From the outset of my quest for information about pain, I was fortunate in having as a mentor Dr. Everette May, the scientist internationally known for his basic research on analgesics. Over a period of years, he patiently answered my questions and explained his own research and that of other scientists engaged in the search for safer, more effective pain relievers.

To Dr. Frederick L. Stone, brilliant health science administrator who, during the seven years we worked together at NIH, indoctrinated me in the politics of the health sciences, I acknowledge my great indebtedness.

And then there are those who lightly dismiss thanks with "It's my job to help you"—the information officers of governmental agencies, universities, voluntary societies, and the librarians of public and medical libraries, especially those at the National Library of Medicine. To them, I say again, "Thank you."

In this era of publishing, the traditional "author's editor" supposedly no longer exists. But I can attest that such is not the case. In Bruce Lee, the tradition flourishes. I am most grateful to him not only for his editorial expertise, but for his prescience, unfailing courtesy, and patience in piloting me through the stages of this book from the book proposal to publication. Bruce and his able and gracious colleague, Nancy Kelly, in the true "author's editor" tradition, make my experience one of being "happily published."

International Brotherhood of Teamsters
National Association of Blue Shield Plan
Motorola, Inc.
E. M. I. Medical Incorp.
American Society for Medical Technology
American Parents Committee, Inc.
American Dietetic Association
Abbott Laboratories
National Federation of Licensed Practical Nurses
American Hospital Association
American Medicor Incorp.
Smith Kline Corp.
Service Master Industrials, Inc.
Loew's Corp.
Hoffman LaRoche, Inc.
Consumer Action Now, Inc.
American Farm Bureau Federation
Federation of American Hospitals
J. D. Serle and Co.
National Rehabilitation Association
Damon Corp.
American Medical Association
National Retired Teachers Association
American Academy of Family Physicians
Eli Lilly Co.
American Nurses' Association, Inc.
Women's Lobby, Inc.
Cooperative League of the U.S.A.
American Association of Marriage and Family Counselors
National Congress of Parents and Teachers
Federated Department Stores, Inc.
National Association of Private Psychiatric Hospitals
National Association of Life Science
National Medicare, Inc.
College of American Pathologists
Common Cause
American Veterinarian Association

Index

213

ABOUT THE AUTHOR

Helen Neal has worked in health communications for twenty years as a journalist, freelance writer, editor, speaker, and as public relations specialist for the National Institutes of Health. She is a founding member of the International Association for the Study of Pain and a charter member of the American Pain Society. Recently she was appointed to the Advisory Council of the National Committee on the Treatment of Intractable Pain. Among her books are *Better Communications for Better Health* and a novel, *The Foundation*. She lives in Washington, D.C.